# Meet Me Where I Am

# Meet Me
# WHERE I AM

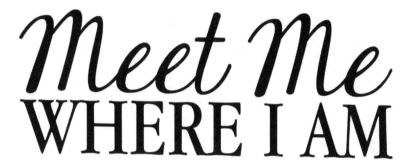

# Mary Ann Drummond

NEW YORK

LONDON • NASHVILLE • MELBOURNE • VANCOUVER

# Meet Me Where I Am

*An Alzheimer's Care Guide*

Published in New York, New York, by Morgan James Publishing. Morgan James is a trademark of Morgan James, LLC. www.MorganJamesPublishing.com

The Morgan James Speakers Group can bring authors to your live event. For more information or to book an event visit The Morgan James Speakers Group at www.TheMorganJamesSpeakersGroup.com.

ISBN 9781683509585 paperback
ISBN 9781683509592 eBook
Library of Congress Control Number: 2018932814

**Cover and Interior Design by:**
Christopher Kirk
www.GFSstudio.com

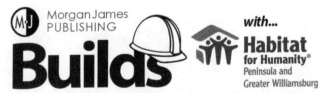

In an effort to support local communities, raise awareness and funds, Morgan James Publishing donates a percentage of all book sales for the life of each book to Habitat for Humanity Peninsula and Greater Williamsburg.

Get involved today! Visit
www.MorganJamesBuilds.com

# Praise for *Meet Me Where I Am*

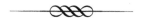

"*Meet Me Where I Am* speaks volumes through the title alone. Ms. Drummond inspires with insight and wisdom, offering useful strategies for navigating this journey with grace. It is an excellent and meaningful book and I highly recommend it."

**— Lisa Verges, MD,**
Geriatric Psychiatrist, MemoryCare, Asheville, North Carolina

"Mary Ann Drummond has kindly shared pearls of wisdom she acquired from her many years caring for patients with Alzheimer's disease. This book will help caregivers and family members understand dementia from the patient's perspective. *Meet Me Where I Am* is a must-read for caregivers of all kinds."

**— Kathleen M. Hayden, PhD**
Associate Professor, Bryan Alzheimer's Disease Research Center, Duke University

"I have had the privilege of working with many who are on a difficult life journey over my 25-year career as a Clinical Psychologist. One of the things I do for clients is recommend a good book to help them through the difficulties they may be facing. A few years ago, I was faced with the dilemma that I did not have a good book to recommend for families and care providers on the journey with a loved one with dementia. I shared this dilemma with my hair stylist. She recommended a book titled *Meet Me Where I Am: An Alzheimer's Care Guide*. The title gave me hope that the book would be a valuable resource for those facing dementia. Within minutes of beginning to read *Meet Me Where I Am* I knew that I had found the book that I would recommend to everyone on the journey with someone facing Alzheimer's disease or a related dementia. *Meet Me Where I Am* provides clinically respected tools that can be immediately implemented to maximize successful outcomes. More importantly, it provides useful suggestions to help family members and providers maintain connections and relationships as the disease advances. I did not know Mary Ann Drummond when I first read *Meet Me Where I Am*. However, I was so grateful to Mary Ann for writing this book that I decided to call and thank her. That phone call led to a partnership between Mary Ann and myself to write a children's book titled *Grandma and Me: A Kid's Guide for Alzheimer's and Dementia*."

**— Beatrice Tauber Prior, Psy.D.**
Clinical Psychologist

"For over 20 years in Senior Living and caring for thousands of people with Alzheimer's I have yet to find a comprehensive book with information, facts, and the possibilities . . . until now! This exceptional book demystifies the principles and philosophy of living with Alzheimer's and opens your mind to the possibilities rather than the heartbreak."

**— Richard G. Seifried,**
Alzheimer's family member who lived the journey

"With an extensive background in nursing, a compassionate heart and an uncanny intuition about people, Mary Ann wades into the deep waters of dementia where many patients and their families are left stranded. Her acceptance, love and good sense are a life raft as she instructs caregivers and their family members how to be aware of the patient's perspective. Whether you are a caregiver or your loved one has Alzheimer's, this little book will help you make the most of the time you spend together."

**— Ann Campanella,**
Author *Motherhood: Lost and Found*

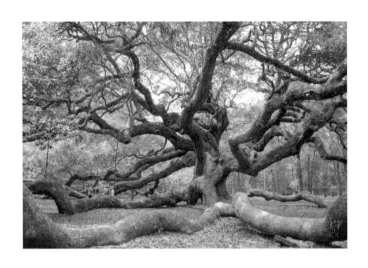

# Meet Me Where I Am

*You look at me with eyes of sadness when I don't seem to recognize you. You see me as confused and bewildered, yet I know where I am and who I am. I'm in my twenties, raising my children, whom I love very much. When you see me hold a baby doll as if it is you, know the love you see in my eyes is real. It is the very love I will always have for you.*

*When you see me recognize a stranger as my husband, know that for me, he is my love. Meet me where I am. Please don't grieve if I cannot relate to where you want me to be. I have no control over the road I am traveling; yet it is my reality.*

*I cannot come to you, but you can come to me. I am like the taproot of an ancient oak tree, running deep into the ground. I am still me, but you may not always know what part of me I am today. Seek me. Seek to find where I am, and you will find a place for yourself beside me.*

# Dedication

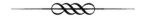

In loving memory of Dolores

# Contents

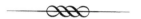

# Introduction

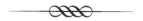

Imagine sitting in your favorite chair at the end of a long day sorting through the mail. An envelope, hand addressed with beautiful script-like penmanship, catches your eye. Inside the envelope you find a card with a picture of a lighthouse and the words *You light up my life* on the front cover. Eagerly you open the card and read the note inside, which simply states: *I miss you and wish you were near.*

The warm message makes you smile, but your excitement quickly fades when you read the signature and wonder, who is this person? The thought of such a personalized card being sent by an apparent stranger is unsettling. You reread the signature several times hoping the name will ring a bell, only to become even more confused and bewildered.

Was the card sent to you by mistake? No, that would be unlikely as it was addressed to *you*. Amazed over the mystery in your hands, you continue to search for clues. There is no last name and no return address, just a simple signature: *Love always, Janie.* It is postmarked from your hometown, so you decide to thumb through the pages of your address book to see if any of the names ring a bell. You notice the name Janie Cass and suddenly you remember . . . Janie is your older sister! Tears of sadness seep from your eyes as you wonder how you could ever forget someone so dear.

This is not the first time your memory has betrayed you as of late. Yesterday you made an entry in the journal the doctor asked you to keep, describing how you feel like a prisoner trapped in your own mind. Your home has become a revolving door of friends and family who come by to wish you well and tell you they are praying for you and thinking of you. Sometimes you recognize them. Sometimes you don't.

Day in and day out the same scenario unfolds over and over again. You have lost your will to argue points of view since it seems now any time you speak, there is always someone correcting you and pointing out why you are wrong. You find yourself desiring to spend more and more time alone, because there is nowhere to go that feels comfortable or right. As you reflect on it all, you can't help but think the whole world has gone mad.

*Welcome to the world of Alzheimer's disease.* Unfamiliar, unsettling, and most of all, unfair! This life-altering condition profoundly affects our ability to remember the most intimate details of who we are and who we were, and eventually will claim our ability to manage day-to-day needs of life. Short-term memory loss is the most noticeable symptom at first. Events that happened many years ago can be recalled with explicit accuracy, yet it is often difficult to recall what happened hours before on the same day. Yesterday becomes today's reality, while today becomes a faraway place that is continuously sought after, and seldom found.

The journey is as emotionally and physically challenging for the person living with the disease as it is for those who love and care for them. There are so many questions that remain a mystery. *What causes Alzheimer's disease? How is it cured? Who is at risk?* These questions remain at the heart of ongoing research and will continue to haunt the medical world until the first survivor is found.

In America alone, over five million people have Alzheimer's disease. By 2050, these numbers are expected to triple, rising as high as sixteen million. This heartbreaking illness has become the sixth leading cause of death in the United States. In 2017, dementia surpassed heart disease in England and Wales as the number one cause of death. Worldwide nearly forty-four million people have Alzheimer's or a related dementia, yet only one in four have actually been diagnosed. The growing prevalence of Alzheimer's is not unlike an epidemic.

As increasing numbers of those we know and love become ill, we find ourselves seeking knowledge and understanding. *Meet Me Where I Am* is a guide designed to help caregivers develop the necessary skills to ensure the most successful outcomes are achieved when caring for persons living with Alzheimer's disease or related dementias.

The greatest teacher is the one who has experienced the subject matter firsthand. This guide is a collection of what I have personally learned from the many people living with Alzheimer's disease and other dementias whom I have had the pleasure of knowing and caring for throughout the years. Through their wisdom, may we continue to learn and grow, while giving our best to our loved ones until the cure is found.

*I thank my God every time I remember you.*

Philippians 1:3 NIV

Chapter One

# Understanding Alzheimer's Disease

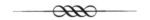

*If I had a single flower for every time I thought of*
*you . . . I could walk through my garden forever.*
—*Alfred Lord Tennyson*

I don't know if it was the love in his eyes or the tear that rolled down his cheek as he shared his story that moved me the most. He was serving on a panel of family members at a symposium I attended. Members of the panel shared stories of what it was like to be a caregiver for someone with Alzheimer's disease. His story was similar to the stories I heard before—but with one unique difference. As he described the journey of watching the love of his life slowly lose her independence and sense of identity, he shared a pearl of wisdom: "I learned to ask her each morning, who am I to you today?" He found that sometimes he was her husband. Those were the good days for both of them. But other times, she would answer, "Aren't you my brother?" or "I'm not sure, but I think I know you." The hardest days of all were when he had to play the role of a complete stranger. Once he learned that his job was to be the person she thought

5

he was, her anxiety was decreased and they were able to better enjoy their time together.

Too often we try to bring the person with Alzheimer's to our world rather than taking the time, effort, and patience to join them in theirs. There are many variables that inhibit those who live with Alzheimer's disease from recognizing current times and events as reality, forcing them to relive the events of the past as if they are happening today. A son who now looks like his uncle from many years ago may be recognized by his mother with Alzheimer's to be the brother she remembers so well. The natural inclination for the son would be to try to convince his mother she is quite mistaken, assuring her he is indeed her son and not her brother. The man serving on the panel learned through his own trial and error this type of approach brought little success when dealing with mistaken identities in the Alzheimer's journey. Paralyzing emotions such as fear, frustration, anger, and disinterest can overwhelm the person with Alzheimer's disease as they struggle to reconcile the reality they are presented with. Trying to force the individual to believe things that seem foreign only increases frustrations for both the patient and the caregiver.

Through various experiences I have come to appreciate the value of meeting each Alzheimer's or related dementia patient where *they* are in order to achieve successful outcomes. My first realization occurred over thirty years ago while working as a nurse on a busy medical and surgical unit. Our shift had reached the aching-feet, can't-wait-to-climb-into-my-warm-bed point. I had just sat down to complete my end of day charting when I noticed her. She looked frail, with silvery white hair and soft blue eyes that seemed to stare into nothingness. You could hear her softly whispering, a repeated call with yearning tones, as she sat in her wheelchair by the nurse's station: "Mommy . . . Come to me Mommy . . ."

She had been a patient on our floor for several days and was well known to the staff due to unsettling behaviors such as yelling out from her room that people were trying to kill her, refusing medications, and frequently getting up without assistance to go "care for the baby" across the hall. Since she continued getting out of bed unassisted and was a high risk for falls, the doctor ordered her to be restrained to protect her from injury. Her wrists were secured with a soft restraint to the arms of the wheelchair and she wore a vest restraint that tied to the back of the chair to keep her from getting up.

My thoughts began to drift between the words I charted and how sad it was to see a human being tied down, even if it was for their own protection. I watched her out of the corner of my eye as I tried to focus on my work. Eventually her constant whispering for Mommy got the best of me.

"Who has Ms. Smith tonight?" I asked.

"I do," replied the charge nurse. "I brought her out so I could keep an eye on her. She wouldn't stop climbing out of bed, plus she's keeping her roommate awake calling out for her mama. If you ask me, she belongs on the psych ward." You could tell by the nurse's tone she was frustrated.

It just didn't make sense to me that the soft-eyed grandmother sitting across from us could have been that much trouble. Overcome by her sad presentation, I walked over and knelt down in front of her and loosened her wrist restraints. I took her hand in mine and asked her name. She smiled a beautiful smile, and sweetly said, "Why, you know who I am!"

Not wanting to offend her and not sure what else to say, I replied, "Sure I do . . ." She picked up my hand and kissed it affectionately, as though she had known me all her life—as if I was someone very dear to her. I stayed there quietly for just a moment as she clung to my hand before giving her a pat on the shoulder to tell her I had to go back to work. She became agitated, asking me not to go. I told her that I had to and got up to return to my charting, having to gently pry her hand away from mine. As I walked away, she started calling after me, "Mommy, please don't go! I want a piece of candy, Mommy! Please, Mommy, come back!"

I returned to my seat at the nurse's station confused by what had occurred. Having a woman in her eighties call me Mommy was a strange experience. I wasn't quite sure what to make of it. As I sat there trying to refocus on my charts, her voice became increasingly agitated, louder and louder, as she continued to call out for Mommy and ask for candy. The charge nurse, annoyed by the patient's increased volume, was not shy in expressing so. "Now look what you've done! She was just fine before you stirred her up. If you had left her alone she wouldn't be so upset!"

The charge nurse walked over to Ms. Smith, who was now in tears; she was still asking for her mommy to bring her a piece of candy. Standing over the patient with her hand on her hip, the charge nurse told Ms. Smith to stop calling for her mommy since she herself was eighty-eight years old and her mother was long since passed away. "And as for the candy," her tone was cold and clinical, "you should know better than to ask for candy since you're a diabetic. You'll not be getting any candy around here. Now if you don't be quiet and settle down I'm going to take you back and put you to bed . . . You're too old to be acting like such a big baby." The charge nurse walked away to complete final rounds, shaking her head and mumbling something about "young nurses these days!"

My more experienced coworker's words struck hard with my newfound friend. I could see more tears forming in Ms. Smith's soft blue eyes. When the charge nurse was out of site, Ms. Smith motioned for me to come to her, which I quickly did. This time she grabbed my arm, pulling me close while cupping her hand around my ear like a little child about to share a treasured secret. "I knew you would come back, Mommy," she whispered. "I love you." What could I do at that point but wipe the tears from her eyes and say, "I love you, too"?

I had been taught that reality orientation, the process of helping one to recognize the correct time, place, and person, was the best intervention for anyone who experienced confusion or delusions. However, it just didn't make sense to do something that would upset Ms. Smith further, especially just in order to tell her something she seemed to truly believe—that she was a little girl and that I was her mother—was false.

I knelt beside her once again and pulled a piece of peppermint from my pocket and gave it to her. She smiled as bright as the sun while she opened the candy and began crunching away. Knowing that somehow at that moment she felt as though she was with her mother, I told her that her mommy loved her, and that everything would be okay. She pulled my hand against her cheek, closed her eyes, and with a look of contentment, leaned her head back against the chair. Soon her grip softened and she fell fast asleep. By the time I returned to my charting, the only sound coming from Ms. Smith's direction was the steady rhythm of a gentle snore. When the charge nurse returned, she sat down at her desk and shook her head saying, "I'm glad she finally decided to go to sleep. Her hollering for Mommy was driving me crazy." I smiled as I said, "Me, too."

While I did not fully understand what happened that night, I knew it was something that nursing school failed to prepare me for. Curious to learn more about her medical condition, I pulled Ms. Smith's chart and found her confusion was due to a diagnosis of Alzheimer's disease. It was rare at that time to see the dementia diagnosed as Alzheimer's. Usually the chart would say something like *organic brain syndrome* or *senile dementia*.

From then on I began to pay close attention to the patients I cared for who had Alzheimer's disease. Most were hospitalized with illnesses unrelated to Alzheimer's, but because Alzheimer's was present, the course of care was often complicated by confusion, combative behaviors, and paranoia. Many had to be either chemically restrained or tied down with physical restraints in order to prevent serious injuries to themselves and to keep them safe. It grieved me to see them lying helplessly in their beds, watching my every move with sad, mistrusting eyes.

As time went on I noticed there were certain consistencies that were absent in other types of dementias. Alzheimer's patients were usually compliant and easy to work with until someone tried to convince them of something they did not believe or until someone tried to make them do something they were not ready to do. Granted, they could enter into some rather bizarre realities that required immediate interventions, such as trying to climb into bed with another patient they thought to be their spouse or trying to leave to go home even though they were very sick. Some seemed to revert to the times in life that occurred in their young adulthood and relive previous life experiences as if they were happening all over again, regardless of whatever else was going on around them. Most could give accurate accounts of their oldest memories, yet often could not recognize their family and friends when they came to visit. They also had difficulty remembering events from recent days or years.

The more I observed, the more I learned, including to expect the unexpected when caring for Alzheimer's patients and to celebrate the successes. I also learned the more I focused on what was familiar to the patients, the more successful my interactions were. If a patient thought I was her sister, I would sit by her side and, as her sister, explain why she needed to let the nurse change her dressing. If the patient wanted to go home, convinced their small children were alone and needed them, I would assure the patient their children were safe and being cared for rather than remind them their children were grown with children of their own. Encouraging the patients to talk about the things they remembered and held dear brought peace, so I would keep them focused on those thoughts as long as they would let me. This type of reminiscing would often end with the patient drifting off into a much needed and restful sleep.

Today's health-care workers are better equipped to manage the special needs of Alzheimer's patients than I was over thirty years ago. Restraints are only used as a last resort for safety after all other measures have failed. Today we understand better how to manage the natural fear and confusion a patient brings with them when they are being treated for other illnesses. As our knowledge and understanding of this disease has increased, the myths surrounding Alzheimer's have decreased. It is not a mental illness. It is not contagious. It is not a condition of the mind that the individual can control; therefore, there should be no stigma associated with this disease process.

Part of our progress is due to an increased understanding of what Alzheimer's is and how the disease affects the brain. Alzheimer's is an incurable, progressive, degenerative disease that causes the neurons in the brain to die and the brain eventually to cease all function. One of the earliest manifestations of Alzheimer's is an increased loss of short-term memory. As the disease progresses, learning skills, communication skills, and the ability to carry out normal activities of daily living are profoundly affected.

We also know that in addition to the destruction of brain tissue, there is a marked decrease in a neurotransmitter known as acetylcholine, which further complicates the brain's ability to effectively manage functions such as memory and reasoning. To understand the function of acetylcholine, imagine that your brain is a large telecommunication network. Instead of cell phone towers, you have neurons. Instead of phones, you have neurotransmitters that carry the message. Without the neurotransmitter, the message is unable to be delivered to, or enter, the neuron effectively.

One of the first documented descriptions of what we now know to be Alzheimer's disease occurred in 1906 by German psychiatrist Alois Alzheimer. Dr. Alzheimer had come upon a patient who had severe memory loss, paranoia, and other changes affecting her personality. When examining her brain tissue after she had passed away, Dr. Alzheimer observed abnormal shrinkage and deposits to be present. The disease wasn't actually called Alzheimer's until 1910 when another German psychiatrist, Emil Kraepelin, first used the pioneering researcher's name to title the disease in the eighth edition of his book *Psychiatrie*.

Researchers continued to study Alzheimer's disease, validating that brain tissue deteriorates as the disease progresses. For reasons yet unknown, plaques and tangles form in the brain, causing neurons to decay and die. In the 1980s a particular protein known as beta-amyloid was identified as a chief component of the plaque formations causing damage to nerve cells. A couple of years later a second protein, called tau, was found to be a major component in the tangles.

In 1994 it became known that former president of the United States Ronald Reagan was diagnosed with Alzheimer's disease. Having an internationally known figure fall victim to the disease increased awareness around the world, with a subsequent increase in much needed research funding. Many promising discoveries have occurred along the way, including a breakthrough in 1999 indicating a successful vaccination was used in mice. Unfortunately, there is a vast difference between the brain of a mouse and that of a human. A new research breakthrough brings increased hope by using genetically engineered rats rather than mice to replicate the type of brain changes that occur in Alzheimer's disease. Since the brain of a rat more closely resembles that of a human there is increased belief that future discoveries will produce more applicable results.

Another new research breakthrough showing promise is the progress made in monoclonal drug therapies. In 2017 at least two of these agents (aducanumab and crenezumab) entered into phase three drug trials with human participants, including individuals who have Alzheimer's disease. The goal of these medications is to block proteins from sticking together abnormally, stopping the toxic proteins from forming cell-killing deposits in the brains of people with Alzheimer's disease. The data thus far suggests there is some success being realized. Researchers remain hopeful this area of study will lead to a pathway of cure and prevention.

A noteworthy event affecting Alzheimer's research was the passing of the National Alzheimer's Project Act (NAPA) in 2011. The act calls for the creation of a strategic plan to address Alzheimer's with a goal of preventing the disease by 2025. Another breakthrough that is cause for celebration is the increased accuracy found in diagnosing the disease. The only way to diagnose Alzheimer's with 100 percent certainty is to obtain tissue from the brain for laboratory testing, which is not possible to do on a living person. Thanks largely to modern imaging capabilities, and also a better understanding of associated symptoms, physicians are better equipped to identify when Alzheimer's disease is the cause of the dementia experienced.

According to recent statistics published by the Alzheimer's Association, Alzheimer's disease is now the sixth leading cause of death in the United States. Nearly 5.5 million Americans and an estimated 44 million people worldwide have Alzheimer's. Another way to put these staggering statistics into perspective is to think about everyone you know over the age of sixty-five and realize that one in ten of these individuals actually have the disease, though symptoms may not yet be apparent. There is a higher incidence of women diagnosed versus men, which is believed to be due to the fact women live longer than men, rather than an indicator that women are at a higher risk.

While we have learned much, there are still so many questions unanswered. *What causes Alzheimer's?* A multitude of studies with various hypotheses exist, but no one really knows why the brain of one remains healthy while the brain of another becomes ill. *Am I at a higher risk of getting the disease if I have a relative who has Alzheimer's?* There is a genetic component to Alzheimer's disease, so individuals who have a family history have a higher risk. Other factors also contribute to increased risk of disease; some of the most likely risk factors include a history of high blood pressure, high cholesterol, type two diabetes, a sedentary lifestyle, and smoking. *What can I do to decrease my odds?* Staying socially, cognitively, and physically active as we age will help reduce the risk of developing the Alzheimer's disease. It is important to keep blood pressure, cholesterol levels, and diabetes under control.

Studies have touted the benefit of increasing antioxidants and following a Mediterranean diet high in fruits, nuts, and low-fat proteins for optimal brain health. An interesting study further supporting the benefits of a Mediterranean diet lifestyle is the discovery that a component found in virgin olive oil may minimize the presence of beta-amyloid plaque in laboratory mice with Alzheimer's type brain changes. The most common risk factor for late onset Alzheimer's disease (after age sixty-five) is advancing age, although more and more individuals are being diagnosed under the age of sixty-five. A small percentage (less than 5 percent) of cases are linked to rare genetic mutations. These individuals may be diagnosed as young as age forty.

With the increased awareness of disease prevalence, we find ourselves grossly aware of absent-minded moments, wondering if it is a sign of something larger going wrong in our brain. There is a question I love to ask when I'm presenting at conferences and caregiver symposiums: Have you ever lost your car in the mall parking lot? I take great comfort finding I am in good company with the vast majority who readily admit they have. Often I find myself in the parking lot, key fob in hand, clicking and waiting for my car to answer with a familiar toot of its horn, as if to say, *I'm over here!* Forgetting where we parked our car is not the type of short-term memory loss that should concern us. Random incidents, such as looking everywhere for your glasses only to find they were on the top of your head, misplacing your keys, or drawing a blank when trying to remember your bank-card pin number are normal events for the average person. Dementia is characterized by a loss of short-term memory severe enough to disrupt the ability to manage daily life functions. We begin to forget if we have taken our medication, when we last ate a meal, or how to operate the computer. And when something really scary happens, such as driving to the grocery store and suddenly forgetting how to get back home, we know with certainty something is wrong.

In the early stages, it is not uncommon to find the Alzheimer's patient joking about their forgetfulness and ascribing it to getting old. Individuals often compensate by taking notes and writing down the details of everything that goes on around them. When someone asks, "How was your day?" the response begins with pulling out the notepad and reading off the events that occurred. The individual compensates so well it may not be obvious yet to friends and family that something is wrong. Eventually unusual symptoms begin to surface, such as the wife who found her husband washing the car in the rain. When asked why, he was silent for a moment as he realized he had somehow made a mistake, then quickly recovered by saying, "Why? Because it's a great way to rinse!"

As the disease progresses, there will be a continued decrease in one's short-term memory abilities while the long-term memory stays vividly accurate. While someone may have difficulty remembering if they have eaten a meal or how to find their way to their own room, they can recall life events from many years ago with amazing accuracy. As Alzheimer's patients reach the moderate to middle stages, the period of life that encompassed their late teens to early thirties makes up the most current memories. Because of this, they are most comfortable when presented with music, clothing styles, décor, photos, and memorabilia that date to the most familiar decade. Whatever the key drivers of day-to-day life were for the individual during that time are often the individual's reality. You may see someone who was once a lineman trying to climb on top of furniture to repair a fallen wire that only he can see. Someone who was once a factory worker may appear to be grasping at air with strange random movements when, in fact, she is in her own mind, busily wrapping yarn around a spindle.

As the disease progresses, language and mobility become increasingly impaired. Eventually the ability to carry on a conversation will be lost and the person will no longer be able to ambulate. In the end stages, the areas of the brain responsible for maintaining life functions, such as diges-tion, swallowing, and breathing, will be affected. One of the first signs this stage has arrived is often a sudden and severe weight loss, even though the patient takes in food, since their body can no longer digest and process the nutrients it needs.

In order to make an accurate diagnosis, the physician will begin by collecting a detailed history of the patient's symptoms. The doctor will want to know when the symptoms first began, what other disease processes may be present that could create the same symptoms, and the family history. Tests will be conducted that rule out other potential causes for the symptoms, such as metabolic imbalances, circulatory conditions that decrease the brain's blood flow, neurological conditions, and other maladies that affect brain function. Computerized tomography (CT scan), positron emission tomography (PET scan), and magnetic resonance imaging (MRI) are utilized to identify changes in the brain that could indicate the presence of Alzheimer's disease. In addition to the brain scans, it is common for the physician to order neuropsychological testing to assess memory and reasoning skills and identify what type of deficits are present.

A wealth of information is available online defining criteria used to make a definitive diagnosis of Alzheimer's disease. The National Institute of Neurological and Communicative Disorders and Stroke and the Alzheimer's Disease and Related Disorders Association (NINCDS-ADRDA) remains one of the most recognized sources for these criteria:

- Dementia established by examination and objective testing
- Deficits in two or more cognitive areas
- Progressive worsening of memory and other cognitive functions
- No disturbances in consciousness (no blacking out)
- Onset between ages forty and ninety

A complicating factor in the correct diagnosis of Alzheimer's disease can be the presence of other types of cognitive disorders. While Alzheimer's disease is the most common cause of dementia, a person may have other dementias such as Lewy body, vascular dementia, or Parkinson's-related dementia. If a mixed dementia and/or psychological medical history is present, it is important to learn about each diagnosis in order to better understand what concerns are Alzheimer's related versus symptoms of other illnesses. In such cases it may be helpful to consult with a gerontologist or psychiatrist who specializes in geriatric medicine to assist with care management, particularly in the more physically active stages of the disease process.

Treatment methods include medications geared toward helping the brain function at maximum capacity. Cholinesterase inhibitors such as Aricept, Razadyne, Exelon, and Cognex are some of the more common types of medications used presently. They work by preserving the amount of acetylcholine in the brain. Acetylcholine is a neurotransmitter required for effective brain function that is often low in Alzheimer's patients. Also used is a medication known as Namenda, which helps to control the levels of another essential neurotransmitter known as glutamate. While it is not as common as it once was, you may also find Vitamin E prescribed, since it is believed to have a positive effect on brain function.

There are a few side effects associated with the medications used to treat Alzheimer's disease, most of which disappear within the first few weeks of starting the medications. These side effects include nausea, headache, vomiting, and diarrhea. On rare occasions the patient may develop an increased sensitivity and experience weight loss and abdominal pain. As always, should any unusual symptoms be observed after starting a new medication or after a dose change has been made on an existing medication, the patient's physician should be notified and an appointment made to discuss the patient's continued medication needs. To date, medications used to treat Alzheimer's disease do not reverse the effects of the disease. There is no visible improvement in the patient's condition when taking the medication, which can cause one to think the medication is not working, especially when signs of disease progression are present. I have encountered well-meaning caregivers who say, "I stopped giving him that medicine because it costs so much and I didn't see him getting any better." What caregivers need to know is that it's what we don't see that is the actual evidence of the effectiveness. Patients on these medications tend to stay at a certain level of function longer before progressing to more severe stages than those left untreated.

Hope comes in the form of ongoing research and continued efforts to identify treatments, cures, and prevention. Until the cure is found, we must apply what we know to be effective and remember to celebrate the successes, as there will be days when the rains fall.

*Tomorrow hopes we have learned something*
*from yesterday.*
—*John Wayne*

Chapter Two

# Preparing for the Journey

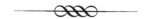

*The road of life twists and turns and no two*
*directions are ever the same. Yet our lessons*
*come from the journey, not the destination.*
—*Don Williams Jr.*

He was a tall, handsome man who appeared much younger than his stated age. You could readily see the depth of his love for his wife of forty-seven years as he held her hand and called her his bride. The look on his face was one of contentment as he shared the stories of their life together. They had their ups and downs over time, but he always told anyone who would listen that she was the most perfect woman God ever made. I met them at a public health seminar, where I was presenting techniques to assist family members in providing better care for their loved ones with Alzheimer's disease. After the seminar, the man asked to talk with me about his wife's condition.

His wife sat quietly as he spoke, sharing that she was recently diagnosed with Alzheimer's disease after she had become lost for several hours in the mall. While he spoke, his wife did not appear particularly interested in talking to me or in what he had to say. I noticed that she was fidgeting a lot with her rings making deep sighing sounds as she stared away from us. As he continued to talk I listened intently, observing his wife while trying to determine what stage of the disease she was in. She appeared withdrawn and well groomed, exhibiting very few signs of dementia other than a general lack of interest in the conversation.

"I'm not dead you know!" Her voice had a sharp tone as she interrupted the conversation with a piercing look to her husband before turning back to me with eyebrows raised. "I know what's going on here. You people think I'm crazy and I think you're the ones who are crazy. I know what you're trying to do to me, and I won't let you!"

It was important to know specifically what she was concerned about. Often we are tempted to immediately console someone when they exhibit such emotions by saying words like *we are here to help you* and *no one wants to hurt you*. Our nature as human beings is to rid ourselves of bothersome emotions or situations when possible; essentially, unloading through communicating our feelings. This wife needed to relieve herself of emotions that were bothering her. This need did not go away just because she had Alzheimer's disease, but the presence of the disease did make it more difficult for her to communicate her feelings. There is a form of therapeutic communication known as reflection which helps to bring out the thoughts of others without superimposing one's own. This technique proved to be beneficial for this loving husband and his frustrated wife.

"You know what's going on here?" I asked, reflecting her own words back in an effort to better understand what she was trying to say.

"Sure I do. It's been going on for a long time and he thinks I'm too blind to see it. But it won't work!"

"Now, honey, you know we came to learn more about your illness, and that's all that's going on here. You shouldn't be so rude to the nice young lady. She's trying to help us." Her husband had made a common mistake that many family members make when interacting with their loved one. He called her behavior rude. This type of approach will increase feelings of insecurity and anxiety as well as cause a defensive response. The caregiver must try to remember the person with Alzheimer's experiences disjointed memories and thought processes that can rapidly change moment to moment. The greatest challenge for the caregiver is to find out where the patient's reality lies and find a place to exist with them, rather than label, scold, or otherwise disregard their feelings. In other words, "meet me where I am."

"She's just trying to help herself! You think you know so much. Why don't you two just go ahead and see if I care!"

At this point, I realized the wife's hostility was directed at me rather than her husband. In the early stages of Alzheimer's, it is common to experience various forms of paranoia, as there is so much difficulty associated with processing the surrounding environment. Your ability to trust decreases and you often fear that others are trying to take control of your life.

Again, I utilized reflection to try and draw out what was bothering her. "I'm trying to help myself?"

"You know you are! I heard him talking to my daughter today about the car and the bank account. He thinks I shouldn't drive anymore, and he was talking about making it so I can't take my own money out without his signature! You're one of those medical people that are going to help him get me declared incompetent. If you ask me, he's the incompetent one. Ask him how many wrecks he had last year!"

I was face to face with a stranger in the early stages of Alzheimer's who was convinced I was there to take her independence away. When dealing with paranoid type delusions the goal is to remember that regardless of what stage the person is in, their short-term memory is impaired. If you can find a way to distract them from the negative thoughts and refocus to something more pleasant, they often forget what they were upset about. You could try arguing your point of view, but it is rarely successful. Trying to convince this obviously agitated woman she was wrong would only frustrate her further, so I decided to utilize a technique known as reminiscence therapy to redirect her thoughts. Once she was in a better frame of mind, she and her husband could communicate more effectively.

In order to have an opportunity to do this therapy successfully, I had to find a catalyst to prompt her to talk about herself and her past. My first attempt failed miserably when I mentioned how nice the weather had been for us lately, and how this type of weather was perfect for flying kites. She responded with, "You should go fly a kite. You're not doing anyone any good here!" As she continued to fuss at her husband and make accusations, I searched for a clue as to where I could go next. The one thing that caught my eye was the way she continued to nervously twist her wedding rings around her finger. It might just be a nervous habit, but maybe there was something more.

"I can't help but notice your wedding ring. It's beautiful. . . . Was it specially designed?"

Pausing midsentence to look down at her rings, she seemed surprised for a moment and then replied, "Yes. It was my mother's. It's been in my family for a long time. But who knows where it will end up, because if he and all of you have your way, I won't have a valuable item left to my name!" I was pleased that she responded to the ring and focused on building the bridge to a more pleasant place.

"I always wished my family had an heirloom piece like that. . . . How old is it?"

"Older than me is all I can tell you. My mother used to tell a story about how my father proposed and gave it to her. It was originally his mother's ring, and he asked my mother to marry him by tying it onto a ribbon and placing it on her Christmas tree." She continued to share how her father made finding the present that Christmas Eve a game and how her mother thought she was never going to find the gift.

"His last clue was to look for the brightest light on the tree. It was a blue bulb, I think, and tied with a little red ribbon under the light was this ring!"

As she spoke about her mother's ring, her face softened, and the sharpness in her tone faded. Her demeanor became increasingly pleasant and she talked for a while about how her husband had proposed to her using the same ring, and other things that happened the day the ring became hers. The reminiscing had been successful! By refocusing her on a fond memory, I was able to help her find a more pleasant place than the paranoid land she had been in moments before.

Her husband removed a crisp, white handkerchief from his pocket and used it to wipe tears from his eyes as he listened to his wife share the story of the ring. It had been months since she had shown any real emotions to him, other than apathy and frustration. He took full advantage of the moment and placed a kiss on her cheek, to which she responded with a quick blush and then a wink in my direction as she said, "See, he's just as clever as he was on the day I married him."

He whispered thank you as they walked away together hand in hand. Several days later I received a phone call letting me know he was using reminiscence therapy frequently and it had helped his wife to relax. I cautioned him to avoid assuming she will always respond to the same memories each time he shares them. During reminiscence therapy it is important for the caregiver to focus on what the person with Alzheimer's responds to rather than what they may wish to discuss.

This gentleman was a caring and patient person by nature, but his early efforts to help his wife had only pushed her deeper into an agitated state, which left him feeling drained and burdened. In working with them together, I was reminded of how powerful reminiscing can be in the care of someone with Alzheimer's. Reminiscence therapy is a powerful intervention to help Alzheimer's patients find their way when agitation, frustration, fear, and/or unpleasant emotions try to complicate the journey.

A good family activity is to make a scrapbook together, including pictures, mementos, and reminders of the most precious memories and special events that have been shared together. In the page margins, write notes in simple sentences describing who is in the pictures, what was happening in the event, and why each item was placed in the scrapbook. For example, a daughter has a father who once played on an award-winning basketball team in college. He was very proud of this fact. She would want to make a page in the scrapbook honoring her father's time playing for his college team. On the page she could place items such as a picture of him with his team, a patch from his letter jacket, a napkin with the college logo on it, or a snip from an old newspaper article about his team winning a state championship. Under each item, she would write a caption in clear print describing the item in a manner that helps the father remember.

Reminiscence therapy in dementia care requires a specific technique in order to achieve the most therapeutic results. We may be tempted to reminisce by asking, "Do you remember when . . . ?" Open-ended questions such as this can cause persons living with dementia to feel anxious and overwhelmed when their brain is incapable of processing sudden demands they are incapable of responding to. Instead, we should attempt to start the reminiscent process by remembering for the individual, leading the way into a favorite long-term memory. In the case of the father who played basketball in college, we could show him the page from his scrapbook. A daughter could begin the reminiscent exercise by saying, "Dad, you played basketball in college. See the picture of you with the team? You look so handsome!" As she points to the newspaper clipping in the scrapbook, the daughter continues by saying, "Look at this article from the newspaper. The *News and Times* wrote a story about you. You are a state champion!" In examples such as this, the daughter would pause after introducing the memories to allow time for the father to process the information and to respond. When she sees her father's eyes light up, and when he adds his own words to the story, she knows she has achieved successful reminiscence therapy time with her father.

Sometimes persons living with dementia tell their piece of the story with body language rather than words, as the ability to use intelligible speech becomes lost to the disease. A smile with unintelligible words uttered, along with a head nodding in positive affirmation with a content look speaks volumes! In a later chapter, you will learn more about techniques such as reminiscence therapy and how it can help you diffuse difficult situations effectively.

As Alzheimer's disease progresses, remembering the simple tasks associated with day-to-day life becomes increasingly difficult. We live in a world filled with devices designed to help us remember the important things. With our smartphones, tablets, voicemails, email, to-do lists, and sticky notes, we head out confident that we will accomplish our goals for the day. We have become dependent on our memory aids to keep us on time and in line. Imagine would it be like if suddenly we couldn't remember how to operate our computer, check our voicemail, or even find our way to work? Life would be forever altered as we know it.

In the early stages of Alzheimer's, a person is usually aware of their memory deficits. Before a diagnosis is made, it is common to learn the individual was suspecting something was wrong but had been afraid to share their suspicions due to worry that someone would think they were crazy or losing their mind. They begin to adjust by leaving themselves notes and reminders of various sorts to get through the day.

For example, I met a lady at a meeting once who couldn't find her car keys when it was time to leave. She was clearly embarrassed when she asked me to help her search for them, and she began to joke nervously regarding how she finds herself frequently forgetting things. "I even have to write a note to myself to remember to turn off the stove. . . . I'm just so busy all the time that I keep forgetting the little things!" She showed me the palm of her hand, where several small notes were written.

As we began searching the building for her keys, I asked her when she last remembered having them. "Let's see . . . I drove here for the meeting, . . . got out of the car, and put the keys somewhere safe so I wouldn't lose them . . ." Facing her, I noticed a slight bulge under the front of her blouse in the area of her cleavage. I smiled and asked, "Where is the one place women are best known for stashing their mad money?" She thought for a moment, then blushed as she realized the location of her secret vault. She pulled her keys out of her bra and said with a laugh, "I knew I put them somewhere safe!"

The meeting she had attended was designed to help individuals diagnosed with Alzheimer's in the early stages to learn more about the disease as well as prepare for the road ahead. She was in the very early stages, but while working as a receptionist she had begun having difficulty remembering appointments and messages. Her boss recognized her behavior as highly unusual and asked her to see a doctor. She had been diagnosed only a few months prior to our meeting and knew very little about Alzheimer's. Just before she left, she took my hand and asked earnestly, "Do you think I'll still be able to drive a year from now?" I wasn't sure how to answer her question. I wanted to say, "Sure you will. . . . Just learn all you can about Alzheimer's, take the medication the doctor has prescribed, and you'll be fine!" But that would be a lie.

"I can't answer that question. It's possible you will, but probably you won't. The key is to make preparations now, so that when the time does come when you can no longer safely drive yourself, your needs will be met." I remember watching her walk away with her shoulders low and feeling like the most horrible nurse in the world. I was supposed to comfort the sick and heal the wounded. I had developed these educational seminars to help people find a higher quality of life as they adjusted to living with Alzheimer's.

Instead, that day I felt less like a helpful caregiver and more like a bag of rocks. It wasn't until I had the opportunity to see the same lady a few months later that I realized education did make a difference.

"Hello! Do you remember me? The one who lost her keys?"

"I certainly do . . . How are you?"

"I'm doing much better now. I've joined one of the support groups you recommended and I've been going through the grieving process, but I think I'm finally getting closer to acceptance. I've decided not to let this get the best of me. I want to thank you for showing me that I had a choice in the journey, and no matter what happens in the future, I'm going to celebrate today." She gave me a hug, and I was grateful for the affirmation. A few months later I ran into her at another meeting. She no longer recognized me.

Alzheimer's is a type of illness that represents loss. It is progressive and eventually ends in death. It is therefore natural that both the patient and their loved ones will go through the grieving process when they are first diagnosed as well as each time the disease progresses. There are five basic stages common to the grieving process. The first stage usually manifests in some form of denial: *Is it really Alzheimer's? Did they make a mistake? How can I be sure?* At this stage, it is common to seek second opinions to validate the diagnosis. Following denial will be some form of anger: *Why my mother? She's never been less than kind to anyone! It's not fair for such a good person to be burdened with something like this!* Following anger is bargaining: *God, if you will make this go away, I promise I will never do anything wrong again. I'll stop smoking, stop drinking, and then I'll be well enough that this won't be as bad as it sounds!* The fourth stage, depression, can be the most concerning stage of all, depending on how deeply one is affected. In severe cases, one may lose their will to participate in everyday life. If someone suddenly becomes emotionally flat, does not care to eat or maintain hygiene, and is apathetic to their environment, it is important to seek immediate medical attention. The final stage is acceptance.

Another type of grief to be aware of is *anticipatory grief.* When we know that someone we love and care for has a terminal illness, feelings of sadness, anger, isolation, loss, fear of the unknown, guilt, and even caregiver exhaustion can snowball, causing an avalanche of emotions. Anticipatory grief is not experienced by everyone, yet is a normal response when dealing with a terminal illness such as Alzheimer's disease. It is often not recognized until various stages of depression begin to surface, such as inability to sleep, feelings of hopelessness, feeling overwhelmed and/ or a general lack of interest in starting each day. Acknowledging your feelings, talking with others, and taking time for yourself are good measures to assist in the coping process. If you become overwhelmed or believe you are experiencing anticipatory grief, or if your symptoms of grief begin to disrupt your daily life, you should seek the help of a grief counselor.

Diagnosing Alzheimer's as early as possible is an asset to both the patient and their loved ones. An early diagnosis allows everyone time to learn about the disease, prepare for the journey ahead, and receive early interventions, including medication. There are two key areas that will require attention once the diagnosis of Alzheimer's has been made. One will be how to maintain the highest quality of life for as long as possible. The other is to determine who will make preparations to ensure the patient's basic needs will be met; this person will usually become the responsible party once the patient can no longer make safe decisions for themselves. Questions will surface that if addressed early on will simplify difficult decisions and care needs in the future. Otherwise, patients and their families may find themselves caught in an emotional tug-of-war when difficult situations occur.

Ten steps to consider once Alzheimer's disease has been diagnosed:

1. **Simplify life as much as possible**

Establish a routine. Doing the same thing at the same time the same way each day is important in maintaining independence for as long as possible. To the extent that it can be done, consolidate bills so that fewer checks are required to be written each month. If the person diagnosed is still able to work, they should stay in their current position until they begin experiencing stress or issues with job performance. Some individuals in the early stages of Alzheimer's disease choose to exchange their work setting for something less demanding on their cognitive skills, while still enjoying productive and meaningful activity each day. Inevitability, increasing cognitive deficits will prohibit any form of ongoing employment.

2. **Stay Engaged**

Stay socially and cognitively engaged as long as possible. Memory Cafés are growing in popularity and are a great place to accomplish this goal and even to make new friends who are going through similar situations. To find where Memory Cafés are meeting in your area, try searching on the internet or reaching out through local churches, as well as the Alzheimer's Association. Seek the comfort of friends and family. There is strength in numbers!

3. **Evaluate finances.**

Is there enough cash flow to pay for current care needs as well as future expenses? The physician can assist you in preparing any necessary documents to apply for disability benefits, if needed. It may be helpful to know there is a special Alzheimer's care benefit available for veterans, and their spouses, who served during periods of war. The Veterans Administration would be the appropriate resource to learn more about this benefit. Are there any physical assets (home, property, etc.) that are of concern that may need to be sold to generate finances to help pay for medical care? Will it be necessary to apply for state assistance in meeting overall care needs? If so, contact your local department of social services to find out the process in your area, and make the application as early as possible so you will be fully informed of your status and benefits, if available.

4. **Join an Alzheimer's support group.**

Your local Alzheimer's Association or office of Council on Aging should be able to suggest a group in your area. By sharing and visiting with others who are experiencing the same challenges you are, you will find strength, information, resources, and comfort. In some areas, you may even find special groups of individuals with early stage Alzheimer's disease supporting one another, to cope with their illness and prepare for the journey ahead.

5. **Educate yourself.**

Make certain you know what Alzheimer's is—and what it isn't. There are a multitude of valuable resources available online. Websites I have found to be the most helpful in educating caregivers and persons living with dementia include the Alzheimer's Association (www.alz.org), the Alzheimer's Foundation of America (www.alzfdn.org), and the National Council on Aging (www.ncoa.org).

6. **Evaluate insurance policies and benefits.**

Determine what insurance will pay for. The costliest part of the care associated with Alzheimer's disease is assistance with the everyday activities of daily living. These needs are not considered nursing care, but rather custodial care. Is custodial care covered in the policy? If not, is it possible to find a custodial care policy that can be purchased? Many individuals think they have the appropriate long-term care insurance only to find that unless nursing care is needed, they are not covered. If a long-term care policy is present, call the benefits administrator to determine what is covered if and when additional care needs arise.

7. **Consider advance directives and appointing a legal guardian.**

Has a living will, durable power of attorney, or health-care power of attorney been completed? If not, and the person living with dementia is still capable of communicating their wishes in regard to advance directives, assist them in completing such legal documents. It is beneficial to review the options with a legal representative so that you fully understand what rights you have, should they be necessary, as well as the rights of the individual appointing these documents.

In addition to advance directives, it is recommended that any individual living with Alzheimer's disease or a similar progressive dementia appoint a legal guardian. While advance directives allow others to act on one's behalf, they can only do so when the person willingly allows them to, or when that person can no longer speak for him- or herself. Cognitively impaired individuals who can still speak for themselves might make both financial and health-care decisions that are not in their best interest. A legal guardian has the ability to step in and assist with decision making when the person living with dementia is causing inadvertent harm to themselves, such as refusing to receive required medical attention, or giving away their life savings to a stranger. Having a trusted individual appointed as the legal guardian as early as possible allows the person living with dementia to be involved in the selection process before the need for such an entity exists.

## 8. Discuss long-term planning.

For many, a time will come when living at home becomes impractical. Where will the person diagnosed with Alzheimer's live when it is no longer safe to live at home? Options should be discussed and decided as early as possible to make transitions easier when it becomes necessary. Sometimes families choose to arrange for continuous care in the home setting or move their loved one to live with other family members to assist with care. Due to the high degree of hands-on care required, others may find it necessary to seek alternative living arrangements in a care facility specializing in the needs of people living with Alzheimer's and dementia.

## 9. Begin recording the story of a lifetime.

You may be familiar with the movie *The Notebook*. In the story, a woman diagnosed with Alzheimer's kept a journal from the time she was a young woman and recorded the events of her life, including her most precious memories. When she was diagnosed with Alzheimer's and her disease progressed, her husband was able to use the journal as a powerful reminiscing tool to bring comfort to his wife and himself. Journals serve as a portal for revisiting and remembering our most pleasant life experiences. To the extent possible, journal the stories as told by your loved one, by their siblings, and by long-term friends that make up the best of yesterday. The more you know about an individual, the more you will be able to "meet me where I am" when the time comes.

### 10. **Create a memory box.**

Revisiting pleasant life experiences is great therapy for anyone, but it's especially powerful for someone who has a cognitive deficit such as Alzheimer's disease. While many items we treasure and hold dear have little monetary value, the sentimental worth of an item can be readily identified by observing those things that surround us. The little brass bell by the table may have a special story that you've heard hundreds of times. If so, it becomes the perfect candidate for the memory box. Photographs representing events from the late teens to early thirties can be helpful as well, especially when someone documents on the back who is in the picture and what was going on when the picture was taken. As the disease advances, the memory box can be used to recapture the special memories and bring a sense of well-being.

The more you educate yourself the better equipped you will be to prepare for what lies ahead. The course of the disease can vary greatly from person to person throughout the early to moderate stages, as there will be a random pattern of deterioration in brain tissue, which creates random results. One person may have a more significant loss in the speech center while another may demonstrate more issues related to their gait and balance. Some patients demonstrate a slow progression while others seem to advance much faster. Inevitably, all will experience loss in the areas of communication, ambulation, and digestion, and eventually the brain's life-sustaining functions will cease. It can be a difficult task for the caregiver to know how to meet their loved one exactly where they are throughout the various stages of the disease, which makes early preparation before significant loss is demonstrated a strategic benefit.

I once had the pleasure of hearing former first lady Laura Bush speak at an assisted living conference in Charlotte, North Carolina. Mrs. Bush shared personal reflections regarding her father's journey through the tangled woods of Alzheimer's disease. She referred to the disease as "the long goodbye," which I had never heard before, but thought it to be a great description. Afterward I learned *The Long Goodbye* is a book by Patti Davis about Ronald Reagan's battle with Alzheimer's disease. Mrs. Bush also shared that, in retrospect, after her father's death, she and her family wished they had played more music for him. Music was something he really enjoyed. Mrs. Bush's words highlight how important it is when planning for the journey ahead to surround our loved ones with the things they enjoy the most, making time together to enjoy whatever those things may be for as long as possible.

*Look to this day! For it is life, the very life*
*of life . . . For yesterday is but a dream and*
*tomorrow is only a vision; and today well-lived,*
*makes every yesterday a dream of happiness*
*and every tomorrow a vision of hope.*

—Kalidasa

## Chapter Three
# *Minimizing Loss and Maximizing Success*

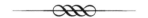

*Up with me! Up with me into the clouds!*
*For thy song, Lark, is strong;*
*Up with me! Up with me into the clouds!*
*Singing, singing,*
*With clouds and sky about thee ringing,*
*Lift me, guide me till I find*
*That spot which seems so to thy mind!*

—*William Wordsworth*

Mr. Wordsworth reminds us how wonderful it is to be able to rise into the clouds until we find that special place inside our mind where all is well. A familiar place that makes us sing and feel light as air. When our thoughts are scrambled and nothing seems to make sense, finding that special place becomes difficult to impossible. Instead of feeling whisked away in a cloud of delight, people living with Alzheimer's disease are often met with corrections and negativity from all around when attempting to find their familiar place: *No, you are remembering that wrong. Bob didn't come home that year for Christmas. Sorry, you're wrong again. Mary was born in 1964, not 1970. No, you're not forty-two, you are eighty-two!* Just imagine how you would feel if every time you tried entering into a conversation you were reprimanded, or even worse, people just didn't seem to want to converse with you or treated you as though you knew very little about anything—including yourself.

Once while at a friend's house whose father had Alzheimer's disease, I observed how even a loving family with the best of intentions can be less than therapeutic in their communications. Typically when I visited, Mathew would greet me with his favorite joke:

"What did the monkey say when they cut off his tail?"

"I don't know. What did he say?"

Mathew would grin, lift his heels off the floor, and rock forward to deliver the punch line.

"Won't be long now!"

I laughed as I always did each time he told it and knew I would likely hear it again before the night was over.

On this particular visit, friends and relatives of all ages had gathered together to celebrate a birthday. The kitchen was crowded and bustling as we prepared to serve dinner when Mathew walked in and asked his wife what we were having for dinner. She told him everything we were serving, to which he replied, "Okay . . . I didn't know." He then left the kitchen, only to return within a few short minutes.

"What's for dinner? I'm getting hungry!" He was standing with his hands in his pockets, grinning at everyone, oblivious to the fact he had just asked the same question minutes before. Everyone stopped what they were doing and looked at Mathew's wife. Her patience was growing thin with the repetitive nature of Mathew's communications. She looked up at the ceiling and after a heavy sigh, said to him, "Just go back into the living room and sit down and stay out of the kitchen until I call you. You wouldn't remember if I told you, anyway!" He stood there for a moment longer, his smile fading into a flat line as he looked down at the floor, then slowly turned away with his head bent low. Mathew spent the rest of the evening sitting in his favorite recliner, quietly disconnected from everyone. Sadly, I didn't hear the monkey joke again that evening.

Alzheimer's caregivers have many reasons to feel challenged and need to be careful not to let their frustrations show when communicating with their loved ones. Remember to respond with kindness and demonstrate interest in order to prevent feelings of inadequacy and subsequent social withdrawal. This may mean laughing at the same joke each time it is told throughout the day or answering the same question you answered five minutes ago as if it is the first time you heard it. While short-term memory and ability to reason are impaired for people with Alzheimer's, they are still capable of feeling and responding to situations the same way they did before the illness. Being called out for something they did wrong is a negative stimulus that typically creates a negative reaction.

We should also remember that having Alzheimer's doesn't stop us from being who we are characteristically.

We lose the reality of current events and times but remain true to our younger self from days long past. Think about yourself and what you were like from your young teenage years to your early thirties. What was important to you? What were your dreams and your goals? What drove you and motivated you to do what you did each day? This is the primary period of life that most individuals affected by dementias such as Alzheimer's disease vividly remember, and are often found thinking, feeling, and experiencing as though they were living it all over again. The person we know and love as our mother or father may have been a lot different when they were younger. Because of this, the person that emerges as the disease progresses may sometimes feel like a stranger.

Two very caring, loving, and most devoted sons had a mother who was believed to be nearing the latter stage of Alzheimer's disease. When I first met Sallie, her personality was flat and she would not follow me with her eyes when I moved about in the room. She had ceased to walk and did not talk with anyone anymore, not even her sons. The most communication she demonstrated was facial grimaces and combativeness toward care when anyone tried to give her a bath or change her clothing. She had also lost a lot of weight and ate very little, and that was only when someone fed her. All of the symptoms were present that one might expect to find for an end-stage Alzheimer's patient. However, in Sallie's case there were a few pieces of the puzzle that didn't fit. She had reportedly deteriorated from eating, talking, walking, and dressing herself with little difficulty to her current state in a matter of weeks. Typically such drastic changes would take months, or even years, to manifest.

Sallie's sons told me in no uncertain terms she had been the most wonderful mother anyone could ever want, and they expected her to be treated as such. The person they described was successful in life, highly organized, and very strict in regard to doing the "right" thing. While Sallie demonstrated a lack of response to her environment overall, I began to notice when walking past her room she would lift her head up and look around. I began to observe her from around the corner to see what other kinds of activity she demonstrated when she was alone. I was surprised to learn she had a little ritual she performed with her covers, wherein she would pull them high upon her shoulders, fold the top down, and form a crease on the folded edge with her hands. She would then lay her arms on top of the cover by her side with her hands lightly grasped together. These actions suggested to me that maybe Sallie wasn't in the end stages of her disease. It seemed as though, when she was alone, she wasn't as flat and tuned out to the world around her as she was when we were with her in the room. Maybe she was depressed, or maybe she was simply afraid because the home and life she remembered was gone to her.

To test my theory, I began working more closely with Sallie. I started by making slow and deliberate moves at her bedside, announcing myself while taking her hand in mine and standing in her line of vision. I whispered little messages in Sallie's ear, such as "You are safe here. . . . No one is going to hurt you. . . . If you want to get up, just let me know by raising your head and I will help you." Upon my first attempts, it appeared I was wrong since she gave no response. After multiple tries on different occasions, and then standing quietly in her room waiting for a sign, Sallie did raise her head up and looked all around. Taking full advantage of the moment, I walked over and asked if she would like to stand and walk to the bathroom. Without a word exchanged, she allowed me to help her stand. With a consistent approach of reassurance that she was safe, and by taking great patience to "meet me where I am," Sallie began to make progress. It took a few weeks before she regained strength to walk on her own. As her feeling of security increased so did her interactions with her sons and the facility staff. Eventually she had returned to the previous productive level of function she had been at several weeks before. All in all, I thought it was a great success story, . . . that is, until the day her sons came to me furious, demanding to know what we had done to their mother.

"That woman is not our mother! You must have given her the wrong medication or done something to her!"

I was at a loss as to what could be wrong. As I walked with them toward the care area where their mother sat, I expected the worst.

"She's dancing!" Her son's face was red with anger.

Really? Dancing? I couldn't imagine why her sons were upset until they explained.

"When we were growing up, our mother always taught us that dancing was of the devil. She would have beaten us within an inch of our lives if she ever caught us dancing, and now you've got her in there doing something that is completely against her beliefs!" When we reached the care area it was clear to see. Ms. Sallie was not only dancing, she was doing the Charleston in perfect step and having a ball doing it! All I could say to her sons at that moment was "Gentlemen, meet Mama before she was Mama." No one in the care center taught her how to dance the Charleston. No one even knew how! But she did, and she loved it! When the music played, Sallie would dance and return to some long-ago time and place, laughing like a schoolgirl while gliding across the floor. At first it was hard for her sons to digest, but once they were able to understand the person they saw was a younger version of their mother—enjoying and experiencing an earlier stage in her life—their anger was replaced by tears of joy.

While Sallie's story ended happily, family members are not always so understanding. Too often as caregivers we try to keep the person exactly as we know them and expect only that person to be present at all times. Instead, we should spend much more time trying to find out who they are inside themselves at any given moment. The best way to do this is to ask simple questions, being careful not to make them so broad that the limited communication channels become too overwhelmed in the process. For example, you may ask the person who seems to be walking aimlessly as though they are looking for something, "May I help you?" The response received to this simple question may be a nod of the head as they grab you by the arm and say, "We have to go." The natural response for most people would then be, "And where are we going?" This natural response has many possible answers, is not so simple to process, and may over-loaded the weakened neural pathways of the person living with dementia. For this reason, it is best to avoid broad, open ended questions in an effort to decrease potential triggers for increased anxiety.

In the above example, a caregiver has gained the trust of the person they are caring for as evidenced by the Alzheimer's patient grabbing their arm and saying, "We have to go." The caregiver needs to allow the person cared for to the extent possible to show the caregiver, either in words or actions, what it is they want to do. Were they looking for children they felt needed their attention, or a spouse they expected home soon? It could be what the caregiver inter-preted to be walking around aimlessly was the person with Alzheimer's way of pacing off nervous energy, demonstrat-ing they were feeling tired, or even a response to hunger. In order to identify what the Alzheimer's patient is trying to communicate, a better response in such scenarios would be, "I will go with you". The caregiver's best approach is one that encourages the person with dementia to lead in communicating their needs, walking with them, allowing time for the them to tell you or show you what is driving their actions. Listening to body language is as important as hearing the verbal words expressed. In addition, know the answers to questions such as what the person cared for once did for a living, what their hobbies were, and what their defining moments in life were as this information may be helpful in solving the puzzle. Once we know the answer to such questions, we can more quickly pick up on what they may be trying to tell us.

Maintaining independence as long as possible in the care of persons living with dementia requires focus on ability rather than disability. The "meet me where I am" care philosophy allows us the freedom to attempt tasks without the fear of failure, standing by individuals to help them through the process if and when needed. As caregivers, we can be overeager to meet the needs of the people we care for, which sometimes hinders their ability to be successful in their own care as often and naturally as possible.

For example, consider Emma, a lovely lady who was in the middle stages of Alzheimer's disease. I had the pleasure of meeting Emma and her husband, Joe, a few years ago. Joe stood by Emma's side through thick and thin and was proud of the way he provided Emma's daily care. He described to me how each morning he started by washing her face and combing her hair, and he had even learned how to pin it up the way she used to. He would brush her teeth for her, pick out her clothes, and dress her. He did this because when she tried to do it herself, she never looked the way she did before she got sick, and he thought she would be unhappy if he let her go about with her hair and clothes "looking like that," as he said.

Once while meeting with Emma and Joe, I noticed that Emma had very little interest in our conversation. She was emotionally flat and seemed to be focused on picking at her nail polish rather than participating in our discussion. I complimented Emma on the earrings she was wearing, and she politely responded thank you, but the tone of her voice told me she had no pride or ownership in the compliment.

I asked Joe what he thought would happen if each morning he allowed Emma to do what she could for herself. Joe gasped and explained he feared it would take all morning for her to get ready. Plus, he wasn't too sure she would be able to do anything since she had stopped showing interest in her own personal grooming. I explained to Joe that it was possible Emma would begin to have interest again if he learned how to practice the "meet me where I am" care philosophy and see what she could do. I spent several hours with Joe teaching him how to approach Emma each morning in order to give her opportunities for success. He was reluctant but agreed to try it for two weeks.

When Joe was ready for Emma to perform a task such as brushing her teeth, he had to introduce visual, tactile, and auditory cuing all at the same time to give Emma the highest opportunity to perform the task for herself. Joe had to approach Emma with the toothbrush in hand and say, "Emma, it's time to brush your teeth." If Emma did not take the toothbrush and proceed with the task by herself, the next step would be for Joe to put the toothpaste in Emma's hand and while showing her the brush, tell her, "We need to put the toothpaste on the brush." If Emma still did not process the auditory, visual, and tactile cuing, Joe would continue the process step by step. After putting the toothpaste on the brush, he would give it to Emma. If she did not begin brushing her teeth, he would hold her hand and help her start. If needed, he would complete the task for her, giving her the opportunity all along the way to successfully take the task over at any time. While this type of care approach takes longer, the therapeutic benefit is well worth the time and patience required.

The next time I met with Joe and Emma, Joe expressed that he could hardly believe the difference his approach to her morning care had made. Sitting beside Joe was a vibrantly dressed Emma. She had chosen a flowered shirt with plaid pants, and her bright red lipstick was not exactly even. As Joe and I began to talk, Emma actually leaned into the conversation to hear what we had to say. This time, when I complimented her on the beaded necklace, she gave me a smile and even blushed a little when she said thank you. Joe shared with me that some mornings Emma not only dressed herself but could even brush her teeth and fix her hair. Not every day was a success, but Emma showed a significant increase in both her personal grooming and her surroundings. Joe felt like a milestone had been gained for both him and Emma.

What Joe learned was how to approach Emma in a way that didn't force Emma to enter into his world but rather allowed Joe to enter into her reality. He learned that we all process information in one of three ways: tactile (touch), auditory, and visual. He learned that in order for his communication and instruction with Emma to be successful, he had to present information to her in a manner that utilized all three cues, in hopes that at least one of the methods would make its way through to Emma's consciousness. He learned it wasn't important what he thought about Emma's appearance but rather what Emma thought. When Emma picked out her clothes, rather than telling her that her choices didn't match, he began to say things like, "I like that color on you. It looks very nice." When Emma put her lipstick on and went outside of the line of her lips, he looked over her shoulder as she looked in the mirror and said, "That's my beautiful Emma."

Previous to practicing "meet me where I am" care Joe would correct Emma's choices, change her mismatched clothes, and wipe away her smeared lipstick because *he* knew Emma would never have approved of looking that way. By doing what *he* thought Emma would want for herself, he inadvertently caused Emma to lose her own personal drive—it wasn't long until Emma quit trying herself, and then eventually lost interest in her appearance. When Joe began to understand the "meet me where I am" care concepts and allowed Emma to do what she could do on her own, regardless of what he would have chosen, he found that Emma's interest in herself and her appearance returned. She didn't seem to notice that her clothes were mismatched or her lipstick a little smeared. In fact, she began to demonstrate an increased sense of pride in her appearance, and even selected pieces of jewelry to wear again. He had very much missed her smile, and he thanked me for teaching him how to bring out the maximum function available to Emma in regard to her care—which in turn, also brought back her smile.

Great time, patience, and diligence are required when assisting a person with Alzheimer's disease so they may function for themselves as long as possible. It is easier and faster to do things for them, but as is true with any skill set, if we don't use it, we lose it. Understanding that not every day will be as successful as the day before is also required. Sometimes with very little cuing, the person you care for will surprise you and complete a task without difficulty. Other times you may find you have to do the majority of the task yourself. Knowing how to best present a task or make a request helps to make the good days more numerous than the bad. When an action or response is desired, present information using visual, auditory, and tactile forms of communication. Practice presenting information in the following manner to improve your odds of a successful outcome:

- Hold the object of attention up so it is positioned in the patient's line of sight and tell them the name of the object. For example, "This is your toothbrush and this is the toothpaste." You have just given both the visual and the auditory cues needed to communicate effectively.

- Put the object in the individual's hands and tell them what they are about to do. For example: "It's time to brush your teeth." You have now provided the tactile component of the message. At this point, it is possible they will begin to proceed with brushing their teeth.

- Once you have given the verbal, visual and tactile cues, and if the individual has not begun performing the task, proceed by placing their hands in position to perform the task. For example, put the toothbrush in their hand and use your hand to guide them to brush their teeth. Allow them to take over in the process at any point they try to do so.

Whether you are assisting someone to comb their hair, get dressed for the day, or go to the bathroom, a consistent approach should be utilized every time. The key is to provide the right combination of tactile, visual, and auditory cues and then allow time at different intervals during the process to see if one's brain has made the connection to the message being sent. It is also important to announce what needs to be done in simple steps versus giving complicated instructions. For example, think of any task in terms of steps on a staircase and present each step one at a time rather than the entire set of stairs for optimal success. Telling the person with Alzheimer's disease to "Eat your lunch" is not as therapeutic as the stair-step instructions, such as "It is lunchtime. We are having chicken noodle soup. Sit here beside me. Here is your bowl and your spoon. Here are some crackers for your soup." As you proceed you are placing the items in their hands, walking up each step with them. See the difference?

By utilizing this type of prompting and cuing you are providing the person with Alzheimer's disease daily opportunities for success, which is important for their self-esteem and overall well-being. When they are unable to perform the task, never scold them or point out their lack of ability, but rather perform the task for them and move on. When they are able to perform the task, compliment and praise them on what a good job they did, even if it means they are wearing one blue sock and one red sock.

If they are not aware of the mismatched outfit or cross-buttoned shirt, they feel as good about getting ready for the day as you do. Just imagine how it feels when an hour after you leave the bathroom you find the back of your skirt was accidentally tucked into your panty hose! Or you gave a great presentation, left everyone smiling, only to find your fly was unzipped! While everyone enjoyed a good laugh at your expense, deep inside you were embarrassed and would rather have not been the afternoon entertainment. When your mother with Alzheimer's comes out of her room wearing her bra on the outside of her shirt and a smile on her face asking what's for breakfast, meet her where she is and smile back as you tell her the pancakes are ready.

There are times when you may need to intervene in one's wardrobe choices, especially if safety concerns are present. When it is cold outside and the clothing choice does not provide adequate warmth, or if clothing is layered with multiple sweaters on a hot summer's day, there is a high risk of injury from the elements. If shoes are mismatched, one heel may be higher than the other or the tread on one sole may have a different grip than the other, both of which would create a high fall risk. In such situations it is best to help the individual realize the need for change in a way that makes the idea their own as much as possible. For example, when someone is wearing mismatched shoes, try complimenting the style and color of the shoes, pointing out how much you like them. The ability to mimic is one of the last skill sets we lose when dementias are present. To build on this concept, use your hands to pat your legs downward until you are patting the tops of your shoes. Then, pointing toward the person's shoes, motion for them to do the same as you speak, drawing attention to their shoes. Have the shoe you wish them to exchange lying on the floor beside the shoe you wish them to remove. Once they observe the shoes are not matched, they may proceed with changing the shoes without further intervention. If not, ask if they would like help to change the shoe. If too much clothing is present, ask if you can borrow a sweater, explaining you are cold. If a jacket is needed, bring it to them, telling them it will look very nice with their outfit and ask if they would wear it for you.

We must also remember to protect our loved ones from societal blunders and uncomfortable or rude public situations, since the average American is not yet aware of the challenges associated with Alzheimer's disease. A good illustration can be found in the story of Amanda. Diagnosed five years ago, Amanda had reached a point in her disease process as many do, wherein she showed very little enthusiasm for her day-to-day routine. She didn't speak much, didn't participate in activities, and showed no interest in her family or friends. After a few weeks of interacting in an environment designed to "meet me where I am" and offer opportunities for success, she began dressing herself and slowly came out of her shell. What was previously thought to be a manifestation of her disease process had actually been depression over loss of abilities. In a short time Amanda surprised her family by sitting down at the piano and playing hymns in perfect harmony. Her family told us she had not played for years, and they thought that she couldn't play anymore.

As Amanda continued to make progress, she started wearing makeup again and had a most interesting way of applying bright-blue eye shadow across the entire area of her eyelids and around her eyes. She also did something else rather unique from time to time, and that was to put her underwear on the outside of her pants. Amanda's daughter had a hard time understanding how or why it would be inappropriate to correct her mother's dressing techniques. She could not understand why she should rather praise her mother on her appearance each day she dressed herself. She told me, "My mother is a very proper woman, and she would NEVER let herself be seen like this!"

At that point her mother walked by carrying a pocketbook and wearing an old straw hat. She smiled and stuck her head in the door where we were sitting and asked us if we knew where the ladies room was. As she turned to leave, she commented on what a lovely day it was, and that she hoped to see us again soon. I asked Amanda's daughter if she remembered how sad and withdrawn her mother had been just weeks before, and then asked if she could see how much happier and interactive her mother had become. Amanda's daughter acknowledged there was a marked difference. I explained it was, in part, because we did not ever tell Amanda her dress was inappropriate, but rather we told her how beautiful she was. Amanda was no longer afraid to interact in her environment and was no longer depressed. She was pleased with the way she looked, taking pride in her ability to dress herself each day. By letting Amanda do what she could for herself each day, her caregivers were practicing "meet me where I am" care and Amanda was thriving. It was understood there would come a time when

Amanda would stop having the ability to perform these tasks independently due to Alzheimer's disease. When that time came, her caregivers would take over her care and do all of her care tasks for her.

After our discussion, Amanda's daughter calmed down and began to better understand the need to allow her mother the freedom to be successful. She frequently took her mother home for long weekends and family visits and helped her mother to maintain her independence by not correcting her or causing her to feel unsuccessful.

One day when Amanda was at home with her daughter, she needed to go to the doctor. It was also one of the days that Amanda had dressed herself and, true to form, had put her underwear on the outside of her pants. She had applied her favorite bright-blue eye shadow all the way to the top of her eyebrows as well. Amanda's daughter had become so comfortable with the acceptance of her mother's disease process that she did not think about how others in the outside world may perceive her mother.

Amanda returned to the facility later that day, agitated and acting unusual in several ways. When I asked her daughter what happened, she explained she had taken her to the doctor's office where a young boy kept staring at her and asking her if she was a clown. Then the doctor came in and commented on the way she was dressed, making a joke about her new fashion statement. Amanda at that point looked down, became aware of her error, and suddenly felt ashamed of her appearance. She had not been able to calm down since.

While it is ideal to allow the individual the freedom to dress and groom themselves, we should protect them from being made fun of or made to feel inappropriate. When necessary, it is appropriate to help them change into more suitable attire when going out in public. When doing this, we should never say things to encourage them to change that would point out their inappropriateness, but rather find a way to make it their idea, like asking them if they want to change into their favorite dress before going to the doctor.

Another technique that has proven beneficial in increasing independence and minimizing loss is the use of visual aids. As shared previously, we process information in one of three ways: visual, auditory, and tactile, or what we see, hear, and feel. When information is presented to us in all three ways at the same time, even when our brain is healthy, we have a higher opportunity of successfully retaining the information. The same is true for the Alzheimer's patient. A few ideas to try are listed below, but you should feel free to try a few of your own as well:

- Make signs on bright colored paper to denote key rooms such as the bathroom, bedroom, and dining room. Be sure to have both a drawing representing the purpose of the room, such as a commode for the bathroom, and the word itself typed in an easy to read font and size under the picture. You may want to take the individual to the sign every two hours while awake, point to the sign, and read the word *bathroom* out loud. This has proven to be helpful in advance of going to the bathroom for toileting needs to help the brain process it is time to urinate or empty the bowel.

- If someone has a tendency to try to open a door that has been locked for safety, try taping an Out Of Order sign on the door with an arrow pointing in the direction they should follow. When you find them at the door, perhaps trying to exit or becoming frustrated that it is locked, point to the sign and read it to them. They will be more likely to walk away with you, especially if you tell them you will help them find a door that works. While on the way, be sure to find something to distract their thoughts from the exit, such as an old yet still familiar photo on the wall, sharing a favorite memory, or singing a familiar song. This will often cause the individual to redirect away from their frustration and enjoy fond long-term memories instead.

- Communication boards, which are available through activity resource stores such as S&S or Nasco, have proven effective with certain individuals who have greater difficulty with speech and word associations. Communication boards are boards that have pictures connected to words. You can point to the picture and the word to help determine what someone is trying to communicate or what a need might be, such as hungry, hot, cold, tired, pain, etc. These boards are helpful, as they bring visual communication and auditory communication together in one tool, thus increasing opportunities for successful communication. They are also helpful for individuals who may not be able to form intelligible words but are still able to read the written word and can point to what they wish to say.

The more a person responds to visual aids, the more you should continue to make signs, post arrows, and provide visual directions. While it doesn't work for everyone, it can make a great difference for some in assisting them to continue to do certain things for themselves.

Opportunities for success should be included as much as possible in the daily environment. Something as simple as being able to fold a washcloth or help wipe off the table can have great therapeutic value for the self-esteem of an Alzheimer's patient. Meaningful activities performed successfully are a powerful aid in helping to maintain a high quality of life. Whatever we liked to do before we became ill is generally what we still like to do after diagnosis, but the activity may need to be modified in order to be successful.

The wife of a gentleman who loved to play golf once asked me if it was better to remove the golf clubs, photos, and other memorabilia from sight, as he seemed sad when he looked at them since he could no longer remember how to play. In situations such as this, it is best to try modified activities that allow participation in a way that fosters feelings of success, measuring how the person with dementia responds. For example, the wife could buy her husband a set of golf balls and ask him to mark his balls, or present him with old golf balls that need cleaning and help him to clean the balls and the clubs. She could find an old scorecard in his golf bag and review how well he did on the back nine. These are examples of golf-related activities that a person with moderate Alzheimer's disease could accomplish successfully. The wife should not assume her husband's response to these activities would be positive. If he enjoyed doing these activities, then the wife should consider keeping the golf reminders in his environment and the activities would be deemed a success. If doing golf-related activities made the husband frustrated, angry, or depressed because he can no longer play the game, then it would be best to remove all reminders of golf from the home to avoid future feelings of failure or frustration.

In the following list of do's and don'ts you will find information that will be helpful in maximizing independence as well as improve your chances of having successful interactions. This list is a compilation of information available from various resources in the industry as well as personal lessons learned.

## Alzheimer's Care Do's and Don'ts

*Do* present information using tactile, verbal, and visual cues. When all three forms of communication are used with simple, straightforward concepts, the odds increase significantly that the message being sent will be received correctly. In addition, the ability to successfully follow the command given is also increased.

*Do* use simple sentences geared toward a specific response. Avoid open-ended questions. For example, asking, "What would you like to wear today?" could cause confusion and a lack of ability to respond. A better approach would be to ask, "Would you like to wear the red dress or the green dress?" In this example, a simple thought has been communicated and there is a much higher chance the brain will be able to process a successful response.

*Do* allow time for the individual to process the information before moving on to the next thought. We must remember to observe not only the verbal communication but all body language as well. If there are signs of agitation, change the topic to avoid further frustrations.

*Do* identify simple tasks, such as folding washcloths, sorting socks, wiping the table, or dusting furniture, that the individual can still do, and ask them to help you do the task from time to time. This is therapeutic both as an opportunity for success and to keep the patient's mind occupied in meaningful activity, thus preventing boredom.

*Do* celebrate the successes, even the small ones. We all feel better when someone tells us we are doing a good job. Compliment and praise are great medicine.

*Do* observe the person's response to each situation, and remember to "meet me where I am" rather than pull the person you are caring for into your thoughts, opinions, and position.

*Do* provide enjoyable and meaningful activity throughout the day. One of the last skill sets persons living with Alzheimer's disease lose is the ability to mimic. Knowing this, caregivers can find simple yet fun activities to do with those they care for, such as singing a well-loved hymn together, playing Simon says, making funny faces in the mirror together, or tossing a balloon or softball back and forth. Activities like this can be great fun as well as great therapy.

*Do not* try to force someone to do something if it is obvious they are not going to be able to perform the task. You must realize that from moment to moment, day to day—due to the very nature of the disease—the brain is battling a spiderweb of tangled communications. Sometimes the messages break free from the web, and other times they become lost forever.

*Do not* scold, argue with, ridicule, or make fun of the individual in any way. Remember, a negative stimulus will create a negative response.

*Do not* continue with a task if it is clear the individual is becoming agitated. It is better to stop for a while and then try reapproaching the task once the agitation has passed. Usually this takes about fifteen to twenty minutes.

When you first begin practicing the "meet me where I am" care approach, it may take a few weeks before you see the fruit of your labor. Be patient and be flexible, knowing that what works today will not always work tomorrow.

Sometimes a new symptom or challenge may surface that you have not experienced before. When a new or changed manifestation is observed, it is cause for evaluation to see what someone is trying to communicate. For example, a person who is normally quiet and shy suddenly begins to pat everyone they see on the cheeks and laughs while doing so. On the surface it would appear they are in a good mood, and most people respond by smiling back, glad to see they are happy and enjoying their day. Yet when we remember that the brain's ability to process the messages of pain, discomfort, hunger, or other needs is impaired, we also remember that our words and actions are not always what we are trying to communicate. We have to play the role of detective and look beyond the obvious. In this example, the person who was patting the cheeks of others and laughing actually had a horrible abscessed tooth and was trying to communicate her pain to others.

Because the ability to recognize and/or communicate pain is greatly impaired as the disease progresses, we should constantly observe for subtle changes that may indicate an illness or injury. Do you notice that after a fall there is now a limp or limited use of a limb that was not there before? What about someone who normally gets up at the crack of dawn to start the day but who suddenly refuses to get out of bed? These types of changes warrant evaluation by a physician to determine if there is a medical reason for the changes.

Another way to help determine if an intervention is necessary is to ask yourself these three simple questions:

Is the current activity hurting them in any way?

Are they hurting anyone else with their current activity?

Is the current activity something new or unusual for them?

If there is no risk of hurting themselves or others and if the activity demonstrated is not unusual for the individual, the best course of action is to allow the individual to continue in the activity until they tire of it. For example, some individuals who have Alzheimer's disease are prone to repetitive actions such as clapping their hands together, singing a line from a song over and over, or making a particular vocalization. While this could be somewhat disruptive if you are trying to concentrate, remember this may be the only action they can complete successfully and their natural inclination is to therefore repeat it. Trying to cause the activity to cease before they are ready to do so may create anxiety as well as a sense of failure. Conversely, if the activity has potential to cause injury to themselves or others, or is a new manifestation not observed before, interventions are warranted to ensure safety and to identify what someone may be trying to communicate.

The journey of caring for someone with Alzheimer's requires patience, knowledge, and love. It also requires understanding since there are many factors at play affecting whether the communication a caregiver sends will be successful. You should not take it as a personal failure when the days come (and they will) when it seems as though no matter how hard you try, you can't get through. Instead, celebrate the successes and remind yourself often of the times when your patience and care gave someone the opportunity to accomplish a task successfully. Also, don't underestimate the value of a warm smile to say, "I'm glad you are here with me today, and your presence has made my day better." That is a great success!

*The time you spend caring today will be a love*
*gift that will blossom into the fresh joy of God's*
*Spirit in the future.*
—Emilie Barnes

Chapter Four

# Providing a Therapeutic Environment

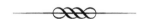

*Oh, the comfort, the inexpressible comfort of
feeling safe with a person: Having neither to
weigh thought nor measure words, but to pour
them out, just as they are, chaff and grain together, certain that a faithful hand will take and
sift them, keep what is worth keeping, and with
a breath of kindness blow the rest away.*

—*George Elliot*

What do you think of when you hear the phrase *home
sweet home*? Is it where you presently live, or is it
a special place from your childhood? When you close your
eyes can you still see, smell, and visit this place with warm
feelings and happy memories? For most of us, there is one
place that stands out above all others as home. Just saying
the word evokes a shadow of magic moments and treasures
lost in time. Imagine sitting in your favorite room, snuggled
up beside the one you love. It's cold outside, but all you feel
is warmth and contentment. Feels nice, right? Now picture
yourself in a place you have never been before, sitting in a

room that feels cold and uninviting. You have no idea why you are there and you find yourself wanting to go home. You begin searching for doors, opening all that you find, searching for a way out. Only, instead of leading you to your home, each door you cross through just brings you to yet another strange place. Safe, warm, and comfortable are feelings far from your reach.

Unfortunately for people with Alzheimer's disease and similar dementias, it is not uncommon to feel lost in your own home, even if you have lived there for many years. The home that is remembered can be so far in the past it may not exist anymore. There is often a powerful drive to return to a previous home and to what is familiar, which leads individuals to a common activity known as wandering or exit seeking. Some people will go as far as to leave their current home to find the home they remember—they may try to walk or drive in order to find it. This is not safe and can have serious consequences such as becoming lost or injured while on foot. It is important for caregivers to recognize the onset of exit seeking and to make interventions to prevent individuals from leaving the safety of their environment.

Wandering and exit seeking is addressed in greater detail in a later section that explores how to manage some of the more difficult symptoms of Alzheimer's disease. In this section, which focuses primarily on maintaining a safe environment, dementia caregivers need to be aware of the warning signs that would signal a person may be at risk to wander in an exit-seeking frame of mind. Such warning signs would include:

1. Staging clothing to pack or keeping a bag packed and ready. A patient or loved one may tell you they are waiting on a family member to pick them up, or that they are going to go for a visit soon and want to be ready. They may even be seen carrying their purse and a few personal items with them when simply walking around the house, clutching them for no apparent reason, but reluctant to let the items go or put them away when requested.

2. They carefully watch doorways and exit areas, and often get up and go toward the door to the outside whenever it is opened. They may tell you they are going on a trip soon, even referencing a place they used to live.

3. They begin to get up various hours during the night to plunder throughout the house, or they may be observed sitting in rooms other than their bedroom in the wee hours of the morning or rummaging through the pantry looking for breakfast when it is time to sleep.

4. They begin to pace nervously throughout the day as though they are searching for something that cannot be found, going in and out of various rooms in the house and plundering through drawers and closets.

5. They begin to talk about having to go to work, meet a child at the bus stop, or go and pick up a spouse or about some other trip that needs to be made in order to care for some family member, or they may perform an act that was once a routine part of their daily work life.

6. They have difficulty finding their own bedroom or ask questions such as "When are we going home?" even though they are at home. They cease to recognize the identity of immediate family members including their spouse and/or caregiver.

7. When asked "Where are you?" they respond that they are some place other than their current location.

When any of these warning signs are present, the caregiver of a person living with Alzheimer's disease should be aware that the safety of their loved one is in danger. This is the point wherein continuous supervision becomes necessary and can be one of the most difficult crossroads in the journey. Sometimes families are blessed to find care within the family; for example, perhaps there are multiple siblings to help share the load. However, caution should be exercised to maintain consistency in the person's physical environment. For example, in one scenario four sisters decided to take shifts each week to ensure their mother was in direct supervision by someone at all times. While this sounded like a good plan on the surface, it involved moving their mother around every few days from house to house. Within a few weeks, their mother's disease seemed to be progressing swiftly and suddenly, and she was no longer able to do for herself what she had been capable of a short time prior. Passing their mother from house to house created instability and removed predictability from their mother's care routine.

Without the predictability of a consistent environment, a person living with dementia can become overwhelmed with the rapid changes and may have difficulty responding to the increased stimulation. The best care environment for the Alzheimer's patient is one where a daily routine is established that maximizes independence while maintaining personal safety.

For some families, there may be only one or two individuals capable of assisting with care and supervision. As it is not humanly possible for one person to provide care twenty-four hours a day, seven days a week, a good alternative would be to hire companion services to be with the patient during the times the caregiver(s) are unable to. When this is not an option, it is time to consider alternative living arrangements such as a residential care program, commonly found in assisted living facilities, where the special needs of the Alzheimer's patient are met. Should you find it necessary to choose this option, be careful to shop around and visit the various facilities available. The following suggestions will help you when making a decision on which program is best for your loved one.

Tips to follow when selecting an Alzheimer's care facility:

1. Ask the facility to describe their *philosophy* related to the care of patients with Alzheimer's disease. If they are not able to describe a specific approach and philosophy, it may not be the best choice.

2. Ask to have the admission criteria explained, including what diagnoses are accepted in the program in addition to Alzheimer's disease. If the program allows a mixed population, wherein primary psychiatric disorders are mainstreamed with residents who have primary dementia care needs, it is usually not as ther-

apeutic as an environment that focuses primarily on Alzheimer's disease and related dementias.

3. Ask if it would be possible to visit with family members of existing residents and inquire as to how their loved one has progressed since joining the program. There is no greater testament to the quality of a program than one from those who have experienced the care provided.

4. Ask what success stories the program coordinator would like to share with you. Most programs focused on quality Alzheimer's care will have readily available stories of how residents showed improvement in their social interaction, mood, and sometimes even in their physical abilities.

5. Observe how the staff interact and communicate with the residents. Do they treat them with a childlike approach or are the residents treated as adults with adult-focused activities and environments? Are staff attentive to residents, or do they seem to ignore the residents' presence? Ask to see the posted activity calendar and see if the types of activities provided would be of interest to your loved one.

6. Observe the hygiene of the residents. Are they neatly groomed and freshly shaven? Are their fingernails clean?

7. Observe the interaction of the residents with each other. Are they socializing with one another, seeking the companionship of one another, or are they sitting isolated and withdrawn with limited interaction?

8. Ask how the facility handles residents when difficult scenarios surface that may be hard to manage. Is their first response medication management wherein the residents are given tranquilizers to calm them? In the answers provided, do you hear techniques such as redirection and reminiscing to bring the resident to a better place of mind? Does it appear the facility provides training to their team members on appropriate techniques to intervene when the difficult symptoms of dementia surface?

9. Observe the physical layout of the program. Is there a secured setting that requires the use of some security measure at entrances and exits to come and go, or does the facility depend on a bracelet or anklet monitor that alarms upon exit but does not prevent the resident from leaving? This is an important consideration if the individual you are seeking placement for has any history of wandering or exit seeking.

10. Is independence promoted with a secured outdoor area wherein the resident is free to come and go? Is there a gardening area and walking pathway to provide adequate space to pace or walk off nervous energy?

11. Observe what types of television programs are allowed in the TV room. Do you see evidence of old favorite titles such as *Lawrence Welk, I Love Lucy, Andy Griffith,* or other similar shows that recap pleasant times from the past, or are the programs geared toward the tastes and times of the facility staff?

12. Last but not least, be sure to visit the facility after-hours and on weekends and evaluate if the program is consistent with what you observed during your guided tour. In a good program, you will notice very little change.

Placing a loved one in a facility, even one that has an excellent program designed specifically for the care of those with Alzheimer's disease, is often a difficult task for family and friends. I always tell family members struggling with this transition the same thing: "If the doctor gave you a prescription and told you that giving your mother one pill each day would help to slow the progression of her illness and increase her chances for a healthy normal life, would you give it to her?" Always, the answer is yes. At that point, I explain that the therapeutic environment found in a quality special care program for patients living with Alzheimer's disease is equivalent to that pill.

When the right care environment is provided with the right care approach, the progression of the disease is proven to be slower and the overall functional ability of the person is often increased. The patient becomes better able to cope with the demands of daily life and finds more opportunities for success, which increases their overall sense of well-being and confidence.

Regardless of whether the patient lives at home or in a facility-based Alzheimer's program, there are several components necessary in the care environment to make it therapeutic. The first component is to implement every measure possible to ensure the physical safety of your loved one. The following checklist will assist you in making the changes necessary in your home to accomplish this initiative:

1. Purchase an external door alarm that sounds when the person cared for opens their bedroom door at night. There are many types to choose from, but my favorite hangs on the doorknob and makes a loud sound anytime the door is opened. This will alert you should they get up and begin to wander during the night.

2. Store all chemicals and caustic liquids in a locked cabinet or closet. Sadly, a gallon of bleach could be mistaken for a milk carton or a bottle of cleaner mistaken for tea.

3. Utilize keyed deadbolts on external doors to prevent unassisted exiting when in the home setting. But remember, it is NEVER appropriate to lock someone with Alzheimer's disease in a room or environment wherein they are unsupervised. The deadbolt is to be utilized only when there is someone present in the home that could safely assist the person cared for with exiting should an emergency situation arise, such as a fire.

4. Purchase an Alzheimer's identification bracelet to be worn by the person cared for at all times. The bracelet provides information on whom to contact should the person become lost or inadvertently separated from you.

5. Prepare a search and rescue kit just in case your loved one ever becomes lost and needs to be found.

This kit should be kept in an air-tight plastic bag and include an article of clothing worn by your loved one, such as a sock or T-shirt, several recent photos that show a close-up of their face, and a list of places that your loved one may try to reach if they were lost, such as the address of where they lived most of their life, a favorite store, the address of a close friend whom they used to visit frequently, etc. The article of clothing would be useful to assist K-9 units to quickly track anyone traveling on foot, and the other items would help the police in search and rescue efforts.

6. To prevent falls, remove throw rugs that are prone to slipping or flipping up on the edges when walked on. Ensure adequate lighting is present to increase visual accuracy when ambulating around objects.

7. Keep hand tools, drills, saws, and sharp instruments such as knifes and scissors in locations that are not accessible to the patient. These items should be used by the patient with caution and under close supervision to prevent accidental injury.

8. Keep medications stored safely out of reach. Maintain a compliant medication regimen. There have been many unfortunate instances wherein someone with Alzheimer's disease was injured through accidental ingestion by accessing either their own medications or the medications of others. Family members also need to become familiar with the medications prescribed for

their loved ones, including the purpose of the medications and the possible side effects to watch for, should an adverse reaction occur. Since the ability to communicate feelings and physical manifestations effectively is impaired, becoming educated on what would be a negative response to medications can assist you in seeking timely medical attention when reactions occur in the patient.

9. Consider the use of a GPS tracking device to wear such as a watch, to place on any car the person living with dementia may have access to, or other GPS wearables designed for the safe return of cognitively impaired individuals should the person living with dementia become separated from their caregiver.

Last but not least, a therapeutic care environment requires an abundance of patience and love. We tend to thrive best when we are accepted for who we are rather than ridiculed or made to feel incompetent for what we are not.

Does it matter if the socks they just matched while helping to fold the laundry are not correct? Is it important to point out that when they helped you set the table they put two spoons out and no fork? If they feel they have done something helpful and are unaware of the errors, it is best to accept that they have done their best and compliment them on a job well done. If they are helping to rinse the dishes, wait until they have moved on to other interests to go behind them and rerinse the glasses in the dish rack that still have soap bubbles present.

Praise, encourage, and support all efforts that are contributing to the routine household duties. You will be surprised by how your loved one welcomes the affirmation!

> *When we recall the past, we usually find it is*
> *the simplest things—not the greatest occa-*
> *sions—that in retrospect give off the greatest*
> *glow of happiness.*
>
> —Bob Hope

Chapter Five

# Managing Difficult Symptoms

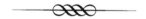

*Kind words can be short and easy to speak, but
their echoes are truly endless.*

*—Mother Teresa*

When we were children, we were often told, "Sticks
and stones can break your bones but words can
never hurt you." Yeah, right! I didn't believe it then, and I
still don't now. The damage caused by an unkind word can
be irreversible. Just think back to those awkward, adoles-
cent days when someone called you a name or made fun of
you in some way in front of others. Or recall a time when
someone's unkind words—perhaps even those of a loved
one—cut deep.

Understanding the impact words have on our overall
well-being is even more important for our loved ones who
live with Alzheimer's disease. I cringe when I hear a family
member or caregiver speak shortly, or without understanding, to their loved ones through frustration: *I wish you
would pay attention! You're just not trying hard enough!*
These words are detrimental to an Alzheimer's patient who

may not recognize their blunder to begin with, though they will certainly recognize the speaker's irritation. They are trying with all their might, but are not physically capable of processing multiple messages, which become entangled in their brain.

Experiencing negative emotions, overstimulating situations, or other uncomfortable interactions may generate atypical or inappropriate responses in someone who is cognitively impaired. This is especially true for persons living with Alzheimer's disease.

How do you respond to pain? How do you react when you are angry, upset, or feel threatened? Imagine feeling such emotions, yet being unable to express them adequately due to brain cells damaged by Alzheimer's disease. You would likely feel frustrated, causing you to respond differently than your normal self. In most settings, such abnormal or unusual responses are called *behaviors*. Merriam-Webster's dictionary defines the word *behavior* as "the way in which someone conducts oneself." This definition implies there is some sort of intentional will in the conduct demonstrated. I prefer to think of the unusual, and sometimes socially inappropriate, responses demonstrated by persons living with Alzheimer's as *symptoms of the disease* rather than behaviors, meaning these responses are a natural occurrence created by the chaos of Alzheimer's disease.

When we are afraid of failure or when we lack confidence, we are cautious to participate. When we feel someone stole from us, we can be aggressive to have our personal property returned. When we feel that we have a responsibility to complete a task and someone is keeping us from that, such as caring for a child, we are passionate to overcome the obstacles and fulfill our duties. These desires and characteristics do not cease with the onset of Alzheimer's disease.

In the early stages of the disease, there is a realization that something is wrong. However, with one's reasoning and memory impaired there is often a degree of paranoia and anger within the individual as they try to process what is happening to them. As the disease progresses, patients reach what I call the *point of grace,* wherein they are no longer aware they have the disease and the paranoias are often replaced with an increased focus on the past and a drive to fulfill past responsibilities. This can cause many manifestations, such as wandering while seeking home, plundering while searching for some perceived lost belonging, anxiety due to feelings of failure, and other emotional responses to an environment that is confusing and bewildering. These manifestations are a response created by an impaired cognitive status that distorts one's perception of the environment. It is good to be aware of potentially difficult situations and to know how and when to intervene to prevent the possibility of more volatile situations. Caregivers are cautioned to remember that what some call *behaviors,* are actually *symptoms of the disease* and not a conscious effort to be disruptive.

At times the symptoms can be challenging to deal with, particularly when the irritated focus is directed toward the caregiver. The most challenging period is often found in the middle stages of the disease. Recognizing problematic symptoms as soon as they surface, and knowing how to intervene, is quintessential in de-escalating the severity of many situations. The majority of successful interventions revolve around three basic principles.

## "Meet Me Where I Am"

Much focus has been placed on understanding what this concept means. To simplify, always first evaluate the person's perceptions, including where they think they are, who they think you are, and what they believe the reality of the moment to be. Regardless of how far off base the perceptions are, establish a sense of trust by acknowledging their reality and using their perceptions as a starting point for all communication. By doing so, you will find it is easier to gain their attention and therefore increase the opportunity for them to successfully understand what you are trying to communicate.

## Redirect and Reminisce

In the care of a person with Alzheimer's disease, the best way to find rest and relaxation is to know how to redirect and reminisce. Redirection involves the presentation of a bold and obvious distraction to draw attention away from current thoughts and/or activities, followed by a transition to a more successful task or topic, thus resetting the short-term memory. What distracts us is unique to each individual and can vary from moment to moment, so be prepared to try multiple things. A favorite song, a picture of a relative who is still familiar, a brightly colored object, a musical instrument, or even a tempting slice of homemade cake are all examples of distractions that may be used successfully.

Remember how effective the wedding rings were for the wife who was feeling paranoid and needed a pleasant distraction in chapter two? By using her own memories of the rings that were passed down from her mother to her, she was able to refocus away from her paranoid thoughts to a more successful mindset. There are many ways to engage those we care for in the redirection and reminiscent process. Start by finding objects, topics, or items that stimulate one's interest, then let the person who requires redirection tell you more about it, even if you've heard the story a thousand times before. Once redirected, add some form of reminiscing specific to the person's long-term memories. This step increases the odds of resetting the short-term memory, thus forgetting all previous negative or inappropriate thoughts. The story of the distraught wife in chapter two was a great example of the success that can be achieved when combining redirection and reminiscence therapy; a powerful duo in dementia care!

## Provide Opportunities for Success

Alzheimer's disease is a thief that slowly robs the victim of their ability to lead a fruitful and productive life. As the disease progresses, it becomes more and more challenging for one to feel successful, since they are constantly presented with the failure of what they can no longer do. By providing increased opportunities for success, the potential for frustration and agitation is decreased while overall self-esteem is increased. Remember Joe and Emma? Joe was running himself in the ground trying to do everything for Emma. He was bathing her, grooming her, dressing her, and taking care of the household. While Emma looked perfectly beautiful at all times in Joe's eyes, Joe's well-intended efforts took away Emma's drive for independence. Emma eventually became depressed and stopped interacting with Joe and her environment. When Joe began practicing "meet me where I am" care, a dramatic change occurred. Emma began to take over many of the tasks that Joe thought she was incapable of doing, albeit not as perfectly performed as when Joe did it himself. Joe learned that letting Emma do what she could for herself was far more rewarding than him doing everything perfectly.

A farmer who had worked in the fields for many years before falling victim to Alzheimer's disease use to wake up each morning at the crack of dawn to ready the tractor and start his work day. His wife was frustrated and at her wit's end; no matter how many times she told her husband they no longer had a farm, tractor, or field to plow, he didn't believe her. He would become belligerent, argumentative, and aggressive through the morning, while he remained fixated on what he perceived as an unmet responsibility and blamed his wife for keeping him from it. His wife learned how to use the concepts of "meet me where I am," which were met with wonderful success for both her and her husband. When he woke up and told her it was time go plow the lower forty, she would graciously smile and compliment him on how well he managed their farm. They would then enjoy breakfast and a cup of coffee as she listened to him plan the day and talk about what needed planting, what he thought the price of grain would be that year, and what they would have to do if the rain didn't fall soon. She knew that when he put his cap on that meant it was time for action.

"Hold on a minute and I'll walk out with you!"

She would walk up to him, place a kiss on his cheek, and take him by the hand while escorting him toward the door. She would always stop on the way at the bottom of the stairs where they had placed many photographs and portraits of their life together throughout the years.

"Would you look at that? It's a picture of our wedding day! You were the most handsome man I'd ever known! And there's a picture of your mother. I think Jenny looks a lot like her when she was younger, don't you?"

For a long time, she found the simple diversion of stopping at the staircase to reminisce over the family photo wall was diversion enough to help him forget his fixation to plow the fields. Once she had successfully reset his focus, she would ask him to help her do some small task that he was still able to do successfully, such as help to set the table or help fold the washcloths. On occasion, he would return to the previous thoughts throughout the day and again attempt to go to work. She would say things such as, "But you already did it and now you get to rest. It's too hot today. We can do it tomorrow." The methods worked beautifully.

While there are many unique manifestations symptomatic of the disease, such as a farmer who wants to plow a field that no longer exists, there are a few specific symptoms that occur in a high number of Alzheimer's patients. The following provides information related to common scenarios you may encounter as well as recommendations on how to best manage when these difficult situations are present.

## Wandering and Exit Seeking

As discussed briefly in the previous chapter, exit seeking manifests when an individual's perception of where they are physically becomes distorted. Due to the confusion of unfamiliar surroundings, they will begin to wander around as though looking for something or may even try to leave where they are to return to some other place that remains vivid in their memory. Often the place they are seeking no longer exists. You may hear them say, "I want to go home." A natural response might be, "You are home." While this sounds logical, it is highly possible the home they seek is the place they lived many years ago. You may find them going from room to room in the house, sorting through every drawer and closet as though looking for some unknown object. When you ask them what they are doing, there may be no reply at all. Exit seeking is one of the most dangerous of all the manifestations common with Alzheimer's disease, due to the fact searching for what is familiar can often lead to leaving the safety and security of their current environment. There are many sad stories wherein someone suffered serious and sometimes fatal injuries due to exposure to the elements when lost in the woods after leaving their home in the middle of the night or wandering onto a busy highway.

When exit seeking is first identified, it is imperative that the caregiver initiate measures to ensure safety. If the option of providing supervision of care twenty-four hours a day, seven days a week is not available, you should consider placing your loved one in a care facility that specializes in the needs of patients with Alzheimer's disease. While the manifestation of exit seeking may be sporadic, one cannot predict when an episode will again occur, and you should never rationalize to yourself that it was just a onetime event, as it rarely ever is.

Even when the person is in a safe and secure environment with constant supervision that prevents them from leaving, it is not good to allow them to stay in an exit-seeking state of mind. Failure to find the place they are looking for or the inability to complete the task they seek will cause increased anxiety and potential escalation into other negative symptoms.

So how do you "meet me where I am" when the person with dementia is trying to get home to care for children who are now grown and on their own? You can try to tell them the realities of the situation, but little will convince a mother, who knows in her heart her baby needs her, that she is misinformed. If I'm telling you that I have to leave to get home and meet my children when they come home from school, don't look at me and say, "But Mama, I'm your child. I'm all grown up with children of my own. I'm not in school anymore." Instead, "meet me where I am" and say, "Okay, I'll take you home. We can go together." Take me by the arm as we begin to walk and ask, "So tell me about your children. How many do you have?" As I start to tell you, ask anything you can to get me talking about something that leads me away from thoughts of my children. The following is an example of an actual conversation I had recently in a similar scenario.

A resident in a care community was determined to, as she put it, "go home and see about my children." She was using her walker to beat against the door of the secure care area where she lived, lashing out at anyone who came near. Cautiously, I approached her, making sure to make eye contact before I spoke. "You need to go home to see about your children?" Her head nodded as her hands reached for mine.

"Yes! And they won't let me leave! My children are coming home soon and they will be hungry! Help me out of here!"

"Well, I can take you there. Tell me about your children."

"You can take me? You can take me now?"

"Yes. I'll be glad to. How many children do you have?" She was unable to tell me how many children, and I could tell that asking her about her children was creating further anxiety. Since she had mentioned the children would be hungry, I used the "meet where I am" care approach and focused on that thought.

"You need to cook something for your children?" By now we were walking down the hall slowly, me gently guiding with my arm in hers.

"Yes. They will be hungry. You will take me there, won't you?"

"I will take you there. Tell me what you like to cook. . . . I have heard that you are an excellent cook!"

"Well, I hold my own. My family especially likes my chicken and dumplings. They will be home soon. . . . We need to hurry!" This was my open door. She had mentioned a dish that I could tell she was proud of. If I could redirect her thoughts away from the children to her culinary expertise, it would be possible to bring her to a better place and cause the exit seeking to cease for now.

"I was never very good at cooking dumplings. How do you cook yours? Would you be willing to teach me?"

"Oh my! You mean to tell me your mama didn't teach you how to cook dumplings? It's as easy as pie!" By now we had walked our way into the kitchen area. I pulled out some flour from the cupboard and asked if she would show me what to do. At the same time, I placed a brightly colored, old-fashioned apron around her, telling her I didn't want to ruin her beautiful dress. The apron was actually an activity aid, known as a fidget apron. Fidget aprons have zippers, pockets with hidden treasures, and other items for distraction sewn onto them. Providing "meet me where I am" care along with the distraction of a fidget apron worked! I had an excellent cooking lesson, and when my teacher wasn't using her hands to knead the flour and water together, she applied her stress toward a zipper on the skirt of her apron, continuously moving it up and down.

Diffusing an exit-seeking situation is not always as easy as the above scenario suggests. Sometimes you have to keep experimenting until you find the right subject or object to distract your patient or loved one. Be sure to look for the cues in what they communicate to you. When you find that one nugget they respond to, continue to work it until they are no longer exhibiting thoughts related to exit seeking.

Try to avoid keeping the focus too long on the thoughts that drove the desire to exit in the first place. Once you have assured them you will help them to the destination they are seeking, you can usually gain their trust and cooperation, as they have already failed to get there on their own. Now you have an open window to introduce something new; redirect and reminisce to a better and safer place and time.

While wandering is often a precursor to exit seeking, it can also be a normal event that should be encouraged. Walking, pacing, and exploring our daily environment are ordinary actions we all enjoy! Persons living with Alzheimer's and related dementias are often observed walking around to explore the local environment just as we do in a normal day. This type of wandering differs from exit seeking in many ways. Routine wandering shows no anxiety, does not voice distress, and has a comfortable presentation overall. No interventions are required for the person who demonstrates wandering in a safe care setting. Rather, caregivers should encourage this type of mobility, as it is good for muscle tone, historically helps one to think more clearly, and is a natural antidote to boredom.

## Paranoia

We discussed previously that paranoia is especially common in the early to middle stages of Alzheimer's disease. Depending on how the paranoia manifests, it can be particularly difficult to manage. This is the only symptom where I have found the "meet me where I am" care approach to be a challenge in the literal sense. When one person believes another person has lied to them or stolen something from them or that someone is out to do them physical harm, it is anticipated they will become defensive, protective, and even aggressive. In the "meet me where I am" care philosophy, we have learned accepting and entering the reality of the person living with dementia is the best way to gain their trust, leading them to a better place when their perceived reality is not appropriate. When the person we care for falsely accuses us of doing something mean or dishonest, there is a natural inclination to argue and defend ourselves to prove our innocence. Yet we know arguing is never a good solution in dementia care settings.

When dealing with paranoia, we can't gain the person's trust by agreeing that their delusion is real, as that would only make us look more like the bad guy. We can't argue or convince them we did not do what we have been accused of. So, what can we do? It really depends on the situation, but the basic concepts are the same: The primary goal is to provide assurance that the object they are focused on is safe. Then we should proceed with distraction techniques to override the negative short-term memory perceptions.

Once, when entering an Alzheimer's care unit, a resident walked toward me, smiling as though she knew me. This is a scenario I have often experienced and rather enjoy, as it usually results in a very pleasant interaction for both me and the patient. I was completely prepared to be whoever she thought I was (sister, daughter, friend) and was anticipating the warm welcome and hug I typically receive in such instances. With all I have learned and know about the care of patients with Alzheimer's I was *not* prepared for what happened next! When we were within arm's length of each other, what I received was far from a hug! She shook her finger in my face and yelled, "You hussy! I know who you are! You're that tramp that's been sleeping with my husband!"

I certainly did *not* say, "Why, yes I am," and try to enter her reality!

My presence caused great angst and emotional pain for this person who thought I was the "other woman" coming to take her husband away. There was nothing I could do at that moment but turn around and remove my presence. Turning around to make a quick exit, I knew that in addition to removing the negative stimulus, someone needed to redirect her attention and make sure she was left in a better frame of mind. Otherwise, there would be a high risk that her agitation would grow and lead to a more volatile emotional state. I then called to speak to the staff present about what had just occurred. The staff member responded appropriately by bringing out a family album that the resident's daughter left with us, filled with old pictures that the resident still identified with. Since the staff member knew the story behind many of the pictures, she was able to share special memories and restore a feeling of well-being in the resident. Soon the resident completely forgot about the "hussy" and was engaged in a joyful interaction, talking about her precious memories from long ago.

Paranoia can surface in many ways. Loved ones are accused of stealing jewelry and money and even of taking homes away. I knew someone who was convinced her daughter had stolen a treasured brooch that had once belonged to her mother. She would see a piece of jewelry on someone and it would trigger her fixation on the brooch and her belief that her daughter had stolen it from her. Though she was advanced enough in her disease process that she could not remember when or if she had eaten, she could still describe the brooch in great detail, including the color of the stones and the inscription on the back. Her poor, frustrated daughter was at her wit's end. Nearly every time the daughter visited, her mother would eventually remember her feelings of loss and begin accusing the daughter of stealing the brooch, begging the daughter to return it. The daughter would respond in earnest, hoping to convince her mother that she was not a thief.

"Mother, I didn't steal your brooch! I've told you over and over, I've never even seen it before!"

"Well, you were the last one that had it! I know you did, and I know that you've got it!"

The conversation would go downhill and eventually end in an argument with both parties upset. After spending some time with the daughter, I was able to convince her to try a different approach. It wasn't an easy concept for the daughter to grasp. She felt she would be lying to her mother if she did what I asked. I explained that the approach necessary to help her mother cope with the fixation on her jewelry was not a lie but rather a therapeutic intervention entering her mother's time line of memory that would help her mother. The next time her mother accused her of stealing, the daughter took my advice.

"Why did you take my brooch? I know you have it! I wish you would give it back to me!"

"Mother, your brooch is safe. I put it in a safe deposit box, because I know how special it is to you. You say that Grandmother gave it to you?"

"Yes she did! She gave it to me on my sixteenth birthday. It belonged to her mother who gave it to her on her sixteenth birthday. And I want to know why you took it!"

"I put it in the family's safe deposit box to make sure it stays safe. Grandmother had the most beautiful flowers. Do you remember her rose garden?"

"It was my grandmother's and she gave it to my mother. It's the most beautiful piece of jewelry I have ever seen."

"I know, Mama. That's why it is somewhere to keep it safe and later we can go check the box and make sure it's there. Do you remember the white rose that one day started having red streaks in it? We were all amazed because it happened the day after Granddad died. You kept that rose and dried the petals, didn't you?"

"Yes I did. We all thought it was a miracle. Mother said it was Dad's way of telling her goodbye. I have some of the petals in my Bible if you want to see them." The conversation between the two continued, and eventually her mother was telling her daughter a funny story about the time she fell off a horse and broke her arm.

The reason the outcome was different is that her daughter stopped arguing with the paranoia, assured her mother the object she was focused on was safe, then used redirection to help her mother focus on a more positive memory. Each time her mother went back to the paranoia, she continued to assure her mother while offering a distraction toward an item she knew was special. This is the best way to deal with the symptoms associated with paranoia.

Paranoia can also be brought on by fear. When you were a child, was there anything that caused you to be afraid? Did monsters ever hide under your bed? For me it was the sound of thunder. No matter how many times my mother told me thunder couldn't hurt me, I would find myself hunkered down somewhere with my hands over my ears, praying the storm would pass. My mother was a smart woman and found how to turn a character flaw into the thunder antidote—she saved it for the stormy days. Whenever the really bad storms came, Mom would capitalize on the fact that I was very competitive and bring out the Yahtzee game. After this pattern continued for a while, I soon began to look forward to the thunderstorms and eventually lost my fear altogether.

Just as it is difficult to convince a child there are no monsters under the bed when certainly one exists, it can be even more difficult to convince someone with Alzheimer's that no one is trying to take their money or steal their jewelry. Your best success will be found when you refrain from engaging in a battle of realities and instead redirect them to activities that are enjoyable.

## Shadowing

Growing up in rural Georgia, there were many old wives' tales that my siblings and I were made to obey: *Don't sweep after dark . . . it brings bad luck. Don't wash your hair when you have a cold . . . you'll catch pneumonia.* Then there was my personal favorite: *Don't walk in someone's footsteps . . . you'll give them a headache.* I confess, I loved to go back and walk smack-dab in the middle of my parents' footprints on our dirt road when they were not watching! They never got a headache when I did it, and somehow it made me feel grown-up to prove them wrong.

While there are many Alzheimer's patients who never exhibit shadowing, it is a fairly benign manifestation and can be easily managed when you know how to handle it. This manifestation looks exactly like its name suggests. Your loved one will literally shadow you, sometimes keeping just a step or two behind, and may actually bend and twist in the same directions you do. It is thought to be a comfort mechanism used in reaction to some sort of developed anxiety. The shadowing itself represents no harm to anyone, and while it can be annoying to have someone following your every move, it is what is best for the patient at the time.

The most common mistake caregivers make when dealing with a someone who is shadowing is stopping the activity before the patient is ready. For example, if we tell the person who is shadowing us, "I need to go into the kitchen and get some work done. You need to stay in here and watch TV until I come back," we may find the anxiety level increases in the patient and other signs of anxiety that are more aggressive may begin to manifest. The best thing to do when shadowing presents is to allow the person to shadow you as long as they feel the need to do so. When they are ready, they will break away.

## Agitation

A man in the middle stages of Alzheimer's was trying to access a box of cookies in the cabinet. He was a diabetic, so his wife kept the food items that would be harmful for him well hidden. But to his delight, he had found the stash. However, his wife walked into the kitchen and caught him red-handed—with a mouthful of forbidden fruit. Concerned for his welfare, she scolded him and took the cookies away, reminding him that his blood sugar would be "sky high" if he didn't stop trying to eat things he shouldn't. An hour later he was found sitting in the chair in his room. He had taken all of the clothes out of his drawers and lined everything up on his bed in neatly folded stacks. He had put on three shirts and was putting on a fourth pair of socks. He told his wife he was getting ready for work, and he said, "You need not worry about me anymore. I'm a grown man and I can take care of myself!"

Agitation can manifest itself in many ways and can be different for different people. Some individuals give subtle signals, such as quietly pacing, tapping their foot while sitting, or rocking back and forth in their chair. Others may let you now without doubt they are agitated with increased negative verbalizations, slapping their hands repetitively on the table, yelling, crying, or other sudden emotions demonstrating an agitated nature. Agitation is most successfully dealt with when caregivers help the patient to redirect and reminisce to a better time and place. In this scenario, the man's wife realized she had been rather hard on him earlier.

This scenario could have progressed to a more volatile situation, because the man was exhibiting symptoms of his agitation both verbally, with his words, and physically, with his repetitive dressing. The wife thought swiftly, weighing the risk of elevating his blood sugar relative to the volatility of his current agitation, and chose to use the cookies as the diversion. Following the "meet me where I am" care approach, she called to him and said, "Well, before you go, would you like to share a glass of milk and some cookies with me? You know I hate to eat alone." It worked. He came out of his room and sat down at the table with a big smile while his wife served him vanilla wafers (better for his sugar level than the chocolate chips he had his hands on earlier) and a glass of milk.

While it is not always feasible to use food as a diversion, it is important to know ways to distract an individual when agitation is present. Maybe there is a particular song they love to hear or sing. If so, play the song whenever needed, and you will likely see a calming effect take place. A foot rub, hand rub, listening to music, or even dancing can often work wonders. The key to successful intervention with agitation is to be sure to change your approach quickly if what you are trying is not working. When agitation is diverted early, the risk of physical aggression is decreased.

Comfort measures, redirection, and the provision of activity that counteracts boredom while creating feelings of success are usually all that is needed to ward off signs of agitation. However, there will be some individuals who will require antianxiety medication therapy to interact successfully in social settings and ward off agitation. It is not always easy to convince someone who is agitated to take their medication. If you find it is difficult to convince your patient or loved one to swallow a pill when needed, talk to the doctor about the various forms of medication that are absorbed topically through the skin. A soothing gel rubbed gently on the back of someone's hand can be a pleasant experience. You may also seek a consult with the physician to determine if the medication is suitable to be crushed and placed in a food product such as applesauce. These types of medications, while helpful in reducing anxiety, may create other issues for persons living with dementia. Many antianxiety agents have a sedating side effect, thus potentially increasing the risk for falls. Caregivers should also be aware that these medications can decrease inhibitions. When combined with dementia, the outcome may range from impulsiveness in some patients to an almost manic state for others. As different people respond different ways, be sure to consult with the physician should the effect of the medication be anything other than positive.

## Inappropriate Toileting Habits

Urinating or eliminating in a place other than the commode is not uncommon for individuals with Alzheimer's disease. There are several reasons for this, including a lack of ability to recognize when elimination is needed and misinterpretation of the physical environment, wherein a chair may be mistaken for a commode. You may also find men in particular urinate in corners, planters, or other inside areas as they would have outdoors many years ago. Women have been found urinating over garbage cans or squatting in closets. Today's furnishings and fixtures may resemble yesterday's chamber pots and outhouses. This increases the opportunity for the environment to be misinterpreted and therefore misused.

The best way to assist one to achieve successful toileting habits is to begin with a toileting schedule. Try placing your loved one on a scheduled routine, taking them to the bathroom every two hours while awake. This helps to train the body's urges to urinate and eliminate around the same times each day. This will help to reduce incontinent episodes, including eliminating in inappropriate locations. If inappropriate urination still occurs after several weeks of the person following a toileting schedule, you may consider purchasing special jumpsuits that fasten in the back, requiring assistance to disrobe.

Another asset to facilitate successful toileting habits is to ensure one's fluid intake is adequate. This will help to avoid conditions such as constipation or urinary tract infections. A good daily routine would be to offer a cup of water every two hours while awake in between meals. This is best to do just prior to toileting.

## Inappropriate Sexual Scenarios

Alzheimer's disease does not stop us from being adults with adult needs, thoughts, emotions, and desires. It does, however, alter our perceptions and responses to what we perceive. This can sometimes lead to disturbing and challenging sexual manifestations ranging from inappropriate touching of others, touching one's self in public, or attempting to engage other sexual activities.

A good intervention when inappropriate touching of one's self occurs is to place an activity pillow in the person's lap. Activity pillows, known as lap-mats or pat-mats, have colorful zippers, buttons, and attachments that capture the attention and help to distract the thought process from the previous activity. Many also have a place to insert a photograph to better capture the individual's interest. They are easily found online through S&S or Nasco or could be made and personalized for someone's special interests. Also helpful may be the use of busy-hand activity aids, such as sock puppets, which become both a distraction and a redirection tool.

If the sexual attentions are directed toward others, it is important to determine if there are any events that typically occur prior to the event. Does it seem to happen more often around bedtime? Is it only when they see a certain person? By identifying possible triggers in the environment you can prepare distractions and occupy interests before the event occurs.

If the use of activity aids to distract and redirect are not successful in detouring the inappropriate sexual activity, hormone therapy may be necessary to decrease the libido. As with all medications, review the pros and cons with the physician to be sure you understand how the medication works and what you may expect once therapy begins.

## Resistance to Hygiene

Have you ever seen what a bathroom looked like in the 1930s? A beautiful claw-foot tub would likely have been the center of the décor with some sort of wash basin nearby. Bathing every night was something of a luxury, especially in homes that were still fed by a hand-pumped well. Contrast our modern bathrooms with granite tile floors, spacious showers, and water-jet tubs. There is very little familiarity to cue the person with Alzheimer's that this is a room in which to bathe. Rather, it is often a place that is so unfamiliar there is an immediate resistance to entering.

Another reason Alzheimer's individuals are prone to resisting care while grooming is the fact that these tasks are personally invasive. Just imagine how you would feel if someone you did not know started trying to take off your clothes! A natural reaction would be to do whatever was necessary to protect yourself. There are other factors that can cause one to be resistant to care, such as feeling cold when clothing is removed or a history of sexual abuse.

When it comes to decreasing anxiety and combative situations associated with bathing and grooming, it is helpful to know measures that have proven successful for others. You may find you have to try several of these recommendations before finding the one or two that work best for you and your loved one:

1. Offer bathing and grooming at the same time of day the individual typically did so when they were independent. If they normally took their shower every morning, attempting to shower late in the evening will likely not be successful.

2. Use verbal, auditory, and tactile cuing before attempting the task. You may find it helpful to show them

a picture of an old-fashioned tub or shower for the visual cuing. Place a washcloth and bar of soap in their hand and explain it is time to take a bath. Point to the washcloth and soap individually, calling each item by name.

3.  If getting into a shower or tub seems impossible due to the level of resistance, try setting up the old-fashioned wash basin at the bedside and assist them to sponge bathe. This type of bathing may be more familiar and a good option on days when they refuse to bathe otherwise.

4.  Encourage bathing by announcing a special visitor is on the way to see them and they should want to freshen up to prepare for their arrival.

5.  Have all items that will be needed ready and within arm's reach prior to entering the bathroom. Lay the fresh clothing out to assist with visual cuing and show them their favorite toiletries. Did their bathing rituals involve applying powder or deodorant after drying? If so, let them smell the powder or deodorant and comment on how nice the scent is. Did they brush their teeth before or after bathing? Is there a favorite bathrobe or nightgown? Including such items in the preparation layout will increase the opportunity for success. In addition to having the items laid out for use, have the water running and temperature adjusted for the shower or the tub filled and ready.

Some family members have shared with me the only way they could get their loved one to take a shower was to put on their bathing suit and get in the shower with them. If you are comfortable doing this and all of the above fails, you may want to try it and see if it works for your loved one. You should never force someone into a shower or bathtub against their will, no matter how well your intentions are to ensure they receive the hygiene they need. Forcing someone who is in a combative state to do something they do not want to do causes emotional harm and likely physical injuries.

## Depression

As Alzheimer's disease progresses, there is a slow and progressive emotional withdrawal. Because of this, it can be difficult to recognize depression versus disease progression. If your loved one begins to exhibit a sudden lack of interest in their environment or a sudden decrease in appetite or participation in activities that they usually seem to enjoy, they may be depressed. The best thing to do if you suspect depression is to schedule an appointment with their primary care physician and have them assessed for the sudden changes. The doctor will know best if the symptoms are depression or disease progression.

Caregivers can help depressed loved ones by surrounding them with pleasant memories and life experiences that are still familiar to them. Old pictures of family and friends, newspaper clippings of personal accomplishments or accomplishments of loved ones, awards, treasures, and so on are helpful aids to stimulate a more positive affect and help ward off feelings of depression.

Another way to guard against depression and decrease

apathy is to surround your loved one with opportunities for success. Sometimes we take for granted what it means to be able to dress ourselves, brush our own teeth, prepare a meal, or even socially interact with another successfully. Alzheimer's disease impairs one's ability to accomplish even the most basic of daily tasks. When we are not able to accomplish tasks successfully we begin to feel like a failure. The wonderful thing about opportunities for success is that they can be fun and enjoyable activities that you can share together.

One of my favorites is to take a regular sized, lightweight, inflatable beach ball and write one word topics that you know are of interest to your loved one on each color. Toss the ball back and forth, or roll it on a tabletop back and forth, taking turns closing your eyes and pointing to a color on the ball. When you open your eyes, you call out the word on the color where your finger landed and share whatever comes to mind regarding that topic. For example, the word *bird* may stimulate a conversation about the various types of birds found in your backyard, a memory of a special bird, or even having fun imitating bird calls. The word *flower* may bring to mind family trips to pick wildflowers on a country road, or due to the sound-alike word association, a conversation on how to sift *flour* may arise.

There are so many wonderful, fun, interactive, and creative ways to provide opportunities for success for Alzheimer's patients in the home setting. Try keeping skeins of brightly colored yarn on hand and have your loved one help you roll the yarn into balls. Keep a small basket of assorted colored socks on hand and ask them to help you sort and fold the socks. Ask for help with small household chores such as wiping off the table, dusting with a feather duster, or placing napkins out for dinner. Once you begin to look for ways to accomplish this goal, you will find it fun and rewarding to add more and more ideas to your loved one's daily routine. Recreational activities such as balloon volleyball from a sitting position, playing charades, singing together, and making simple crafts such as construction paper cards are also quite helpful tools.

I found it interesting to learn one of the last motor skills we lose as the disease progresses is the ability to mimic. I have had a lot of fun engaging in face-making contests and playing Simon says. It is not uncommon for someone who can no longer carry an intelligible conversation to still be able to participate in such basic activities. Be willing to explore and try new things to determine what your loved one responds to and seems to enjoy the most. This will certainly give you a greater chance of success in dealing with the daily activity needs of your loved one.

For some individuals, activity therapy alone will not be enough to break the depression cycle. In such cases, physicians may prescribe certain antidepressant medications to improve the overall affect and interest level. It is important to know what the desired effects and potential side effects are of any medications prescribed, especially for someone who has difficulty communicating their needs. Read the drug information sheet and discuss concerns with your loved one's physician so you are able to recognize side effects and adverse reactions, should they occur.

A caregiver's reality often revolves around the task that has to be completed, when it needs to be done, and what should not be done: *It's time to eat! You need to take a bath now! It's time to go to bed! We have to get ready to go the doctor now! You can't do that! You can't go there!* While all of this may be true, the Alzheimer's patient often has different realities that change from moment to moment: *I already ate! I don't need a bath! I can't go to bed because it's time to go to work! Don't tell me what I can and can't do!* With such diversity between the caregiver and the person cared for it is easy to see why conflict and frustration often occur.

To facilitate successful care, we must be willing to stand down, replace our schedules and mandates with whatever place and time we find our loved one to be in, and accept their reality as our own. When they refuse to eat their supper, telling you they have already eaten, try saying something like this: *I know you have already eaten, but I don't want to eat alone. . . . Would you mind eating just a little with me?* This is how we walk beside our loved ones, gently guiding them through tangled thoughts and altered realities, to better places where life may be lived and enjoyed to the fullest extent possible.

> *Alone we can do so little; together we can do so much.*
> —Helen Keller

## Chapter Six
# *Caring for the Caregiver*

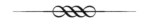

*What lies behind us, and what lies before us are*
*tiny matters, compared to what lies within us.*
—Ralph Waldo Emerson

I wonder if Mr. Emerson might have been thinking of someone he knew who was memory impaired when he wrote the above passage, as it reflects so well what we need to remember regarding our loved ones with Alzheimer's disease. We must always seek what lies within and bring out the best of whatever we find; we must make the most of the day at hand. Celebrating the good days is often all we as caregivers have to give us courage to make it through the bad ones.

As a nurse, I have held many hands and wiped many tears throughout the years during times of grief and loss. By far, some of the hardest tears to wipe away have been tears of the ones left behind while their loved one progressed through the Alzheimer's journey. The person they know and love looks normal and healthy on the outside but all of the things that made them who they were inside seem missing or changed. Some days they find a way to join their loved one in their journey while others they are left behind, feeling forgotten and alone.

At times my own tears have fallen while working with family members and caregivers learning to cope with the loss that Alzheimer's brings. I have had the opportunity to meet some very special people along the way who have touched my heart with their love and dedication. One of my favorites will always be Mrs. Green. She was the poster child for how unconditional love, perseverance, and understanding can be the best medicine for someone living with Alzheimer's disease. I know she is somewhere in heaven today with many stars in her crown.

Her husband, Mr. Green, was a resident of an assisted living community that specialized in Alzheimer's care. He was in moderate to advanced stages and had reached a point in the disease process where he did not recognize many of his friends and family. He was still able to dress himself and took great pride in his appearance, showing a preference for the styles popular in the 1930s. Every morning he would wake up with a youthful twinkle in his aging eyes and quickly make himself ready for the day with anticipation that *she* would soon arrive. You see, he didn't know that he was married anymore, but he knew he had a sweetheart who came to see him every day.

Mrs. Green was so punctual that I knew the minute I spotted her each morning it was ten o'clock. With her silvery hair neatly curled, wearing a pearl necklace and matching earrings, she always looked beautiful and elegant. It was a joy to watch Mr. Green's eyes when he first saw her each day. He looked like a schoolboy staring at the most gorgeous girl he had ever seen. His cheeks blushed with rosy pink hues each time she took him by the hand and walked with him to the couch in the common area where they would sit for hours and talk and laugh. The really special part is how Mrs. Green managed to keep their love alive. She never tried to talk about their life together, their children, or the things that he could no longer remember. Instead, she acted as though she was his "girl" who came to visit. They would take long walks holding hands, enjoying the garden or sharing an ice cream cone. All the while she knew he was working up his courage to steel a kiss from his sweetheart before she left. And he did, every day.

For nearly two years the staff witnessed their courtship continue with the eagerness and innocence of young love. Once I asked her what it was like for her. She told me how her heart ached to hold the man she knew and loved as her husband, but she took comfort knowing she could still catch his eye. She shared with me the reason she always wore her pearls; he had given them to her long ago and always liked to see her wear them. Though there were many days she really did not feel like dressing up or putting on her makeup, she wanted to look her best for him. "Some days he thinks he's meeting me for the first time, but he always seems to fall in love with me before the day is over. To tell you the truth, that part's not so bad!"

One Valentine's Day the facility hosted a sweetheart ball. I happened to be there that day and noticed Mr. Green was sitting alone on the couch watching the doorway, likely looking for Mrs. Green, who had not yet arrived. The music was playing and the residents were having a wonderful time dancing with staff and family members. I asked him to dance with me, and though hesitant at first, he accepted my invitation. He was a graceful dancer and I complimented him on how well he danced. This made his soft cheeks blush, and I laughed while telling him once again what a great dancer he was, which proved to be a great mistake on my part. I failed to realize I wasn't dancing with an eighty-year-old man with Alzheimer's disease; rather, I was dancing with a very young man whose self-esteem was fragile. In no way did I intend to make him feel like I was laughing at him, but that is how he took it. He immediately stopped dancing, looked down at his feet with a confused and embarrassed expression, and left the party to go to his room.

About that time, Mrs. Green arrived. I told her what happened and expressed concern for the fact he had been upset. Putting her hand on mine she said with great confidence, "Don't worry, honey, his sweetheart is here now and I'll have him out dancing up a storm!" She was right. Within minutes he was back on the dance floor, waltzing with his bride. The young man whose confidence was shaken earlier had completely recovered and his joy was obvious as he waltzed with the love of his life.

Two months later, tragedy struck and Mrs. Green lost her life to a sudden illness. Mr. Green waited each day for her to visit, watching the doorway, pacing slowly as evening fell. Over the next few days when she failed to show up, he was so grief stricken that he began sleeping in late, refusing to get dressed, and he lost all interest in participating in daily activities. The twinkle in his eye was gone. When he did come out of his room he would sit quietly on the sofa where they use to visit, staring at the wall as though watching something no one else could see. Though he had been highly functioning with no signs of the end-stage disease process previous to his wife's passing, he joined her within a few short weeks thereafter.

I know that somewhere Mr. and Mrs. Green are together. She found a way to reach beyond the disease and find the best of what was within her husband. She had learned how to "meet me where I am," and though it meant no longer being recognized as Mr. Green's wife, she found a place for herself beside him.

There are so many reasons for family members and caregivers of Alzheimer's patients to feel sadness, but perhaps none are as great as the pain of not being remembered. Some will know what it is like to be treated as a total stranger by the person they have shared their life and bed with for many years. Others will experience the heartbreak of having a beloved mother or father stare at them through empty eyes as though they aren't even there. While not everyone who has Alzheimer's disease will experience memory deficits to this degree, the majority will eventually have issues recognizing loved ones at some point.

Many years ago when my Aunt Winnie was first diagnosed, she still knew who we were and welcomed our visits. She had always had a witty sense of humor and could easily make us laugh with the playful way she compensated for her memory loss. Our first challenge came when the police called to let us know they needed someone to pick Aunt Winnie up from the station. We were shocked to learn she had caused over twenty traffic incidents in the past six months, including the event of the day where she drove off the road onto the sidewalk, hitting a bicyclist. who was thankfully, unharmed. She didn't seem to mind when we took her driver's license away, and even joked about how much fun it would be to be chauffeured around. As her disease progressed, she would often ask questions such as, "Now whose daughter are you?" or "Who did you marry?" For the most part she would still recognize those of us who were closest to her. She eventually reached a point that she could only remember her children. The rest of us had been forgotten.

Though it seemed the last three decades of her life were erased, she remembered with explicit detail the stories of her youth. You could ask her about a story regarding one of her and Granny's escapades, and she could tell you everything, including what they were wearing and whom they were with. I loved to hear her tell the story about the day she and Granny had gone to the fair. They wanted new dresses to wear but could not afford them, so they made beautiful dresses out of crepe paper. They had a wonderful time until a rain storm came and ruined their beautiful skirts, washing the crepe paper away! Aunt Winnie giggled like a schoolgirl each time she described how they had to walk home wearing nothing but their petticoats.

She was my favorite aunt, and I remember feeling that she was lost to me. She didn't know who I was. I remember trying to tell her that I was the daughter of Sallie, who was the daughter of her sister Delores. Inevitably she would think that I was my mother, and then there would be a few moments of joy—at least then we would talk, and I would grasp a hint of her old personality. I wish I knew then what I know now regarding reaching beyond the disease and finding the person I knew and loved deep inside. Granted, it might have been a younger version of Aunt Winnie that I found, but it still would have been that dear, sweet woman I missed so much.

Alzheimer's disease affects our ability to remember the recent past, but it does not erase all life experiences. Here's an exercise that will help you to better understand this point: Think about everything that makes you who you are . . . the people in your life, your home, your job, etc. Compare the you of today to who you were twenty years ago. How many changes have occurred? Now imagine all of your memories for the last twenty years have been erased. Someone who looks a lot like your father approaches you and tells you that he is your son. The place where you live is filled with pictures and mementos that seem familiar, but you cannot recall exactly where they came from. A man whom you are certain you have never seen before approaches you and gives you a kiss on the cheek. When you seem startled by his actions, he puts his hand on your shoulder and tells you, "Don't be afraid. It's me, your husband." This is a small snapshot of the journey that is Alzheimer's disease. Some family members have told me in moments of grief, "That woman is not my mother!" or "My husband is dead inside and all that is left is an empty shell!"

Because so much around them is unfamiliar, it is common for the person with Alzheimer's to withdraw and lose interest in the world around them. The emotions of love and affection become absent from visits with family members. Many people living with Alzheimer's will lose the ability to recognize their closest family members. As people grow older, they tend to resemble other family members in the aging process. An aging sister may resemble their mother while a now grown son is the exact image of his father thirty years ago. Where most of us make our mistake is when we sharply negate the reality of the person cared for and attempt to bring them to our place and time: *No mother, I'm not your uncle Joe, I'm your son Mathew. Don't you remember me? Dad, it's your daughter. . . . Why do you keep calling me Sara? Sara is your sister!* We do this because of our own pain and feelings of loss and a desire to be remembered for who we really are.

Some caregivers have naturally grasped how important it is to ascertain where the patient's view of the moment is, rather than assuming they are in the same place and time together. A young man by the name of Joel shared his story with me when I was helping to open an assisted living facility in Southport, North Carolina. Joel had no formal training but had learned what it meant to really "meet me where I am" at any given moment in order to support his grandfather—and it led to a restored and rich relationship between himself and his grandfather. I asked him to come and share his story with a class of new caregivers I was training.

When Joel's grandfather was diagnosed with dementia, he began documenting the journey via photography.

Throughout the course of his project, Joel began to get to know his grandfather in a whole new dimension. He shared with our class how it used to grieve him deeply to spend time with his grandfather and not be recognized as his grandson any longer. Joel and his grandfather had been very close, and he felt as though he had lost both a mentor and a father figure. As time went on, something new and wonderful began to happen. Joel began to know his grandfather in a whole new light. Joel shared that "I lost a grandpa, but I gained a friend."

Joel would listen for hours as his grandfather told him all about his life as an immigrant who came to America to make a better life for his family. He never knew the feisty, streetwise young man that his grandpa introduced him to when they visited together, but he did recognize the emotion in his grandpa's eyes when his grandpa thanked Joel for spending time with him, and for listening to his stories. It takes courage to reach beyond the familiarity of the relationship you shared with your loved one before they became ill. Some will never know the incredible pain associated with not being remembered, others will eventually relate to what it feels like to be forgotten. What we have to remember is that we are not completely lost to them if we find a way, as Joel did, to enter the time and place where they are very much alive and well.

For a husband, wife, sister, brother, son, or daughter to interact with a loved one in a role other than what is real is difficult at best. Yet when a daughter is willing to accept her mother's belief that she is actually her mother's sister, the reward lies in knowing her mother is experiencing the warmth and comfort that comes from visiting with someone she loves and remembers. The joy experienced during such times is far more fulfilling than the emptiness and frustration brought on by trying to convince someone you are not the person they think you are. On special days, you may find that when you visit with her as her sister, she talks to you about her little girl, asking if she is all right and worrying if she has had her dinner yet. That's when you feel the tears sting your eyes because you know it is you she is remembering. Continuing to be her sister, you take her hand and assure her that her daughter is safe and knows how much she cares.

When I was a young girl, my grandmother had a saying that provided comfort in times of trouble. She would put her arms around me and say, "This too shall pass." Throughout the years, her words have continued to strengthen me when I needed it most. We develop many ways to manage life's ups and downs and to help us find the light at the end of the tunnel. Still, there are times when something so horrific happens, all of our coping skills combined cannot calm the storm within. When this occurs, it can be difficult to admit we need help.

This is especially true of caregivers who reach their limits in what they can personally provide. In order to avoid feelings of failure, many will deny they are becoming fatigued and begin pushing themselves even harder. Eventually, continued patterns of lost sleep combined with the emotional drain of being a constant caregiver will take their toll on the strongest of individuals. If you are not careful, you may find yourself with little left to give anyone. It is important you protect yourself from caregiver burnout and come to terms with the fact that sooner or later you will need someone to help you. To ensure you remain healthy emotionally, physically, and spiritually when acting in the role of the primary caregiver for someone with Alzheimer's disease, you will also need to give yourself permission to take time for yourself when needed. You may find someone in the family who can give you scheduled breaks or hire a caregiver from a reputable agency if family is not an option.

An additional measure caregivers should consider to help take care of themselves is to join an Alzheimer's support group, as previously recommended. You are not alone in the journey you are traveling. Sharing your journey with others who understand and relate to your specific situation can be very comforting. You may also discover that by sharing your story you are able to help others who are experiencing the same emotions, obstacles, and challenges as you are. Support groups typically offer information regarding community resources and ongoing educational opportunities related to the care of Alzheimer's disease. Your local chapter of the Alzheimer's Association is an excellent resource to help identify relevant groups in your area.

Establishing a care routine that supports a healthy and therapeutic environment is equally beneficial for the caregiver and the person cared for. Studies indicate this type of structure helps to slow the progression of the disease. It also helps to maximize opportunities for successful interactions, thus decreasing care-related stress. You may find it useful to create a written plan of your daily routine and schedule, placing it in a common area for all to see, such as on the refrigerator. The care plan should outline all tasks involved throughout the day, including the time the person cared for usually wakes up, eats their meals, takes a nap, etc. Include at least one cognitive, physical, and spiritual activity daily to be conducted at times and a sequence that are consistent each day. A schedule for toileting every two hours while awake, complemented by hydration every two hours, to ensure appropriate bowel and bladder functions are maintained would be necessary for a successful care plan. Another benefit of a written care plan is that it provides information for others to follow when you need a break. By providing the same care at the same time and the same way you do, respite caregivers will be better equipped for care success. When preparing a plan of care, consider the following recommendations, some of which have been made in previous chapters but are summarized again below:

1. Are there any triggers that you know upset your loved one or patient with Alzheimer's? If so, be sure to note what the triggers are. For example, if you know your loved one will get out of bed if the light is turned off, it would be important to note this in the bedtime section of your care plan.

2. Consider the routine and habits a person has followed for most of their life, particularly in their late teens to early forties, when identifying what time you will assign to any item. It is unlikely they will adjust to a schedule

they are not familiar with. For example, if your mother never got out of bed before 10 a.m., do not think you will be successful trying to get her up at 8 a.m.

3. Become as familiar as possible with what was going on in your loved one's life in their early adult years. Memories from the long-term past are the ones that last the longest. Use this information in the notes sections to flag activities that your loved one will most relate to. For example, a schoolteacher may enjoy "grading" math papers, a housewife may enjoy "folding laundry," and a farmer may enjoy "planning the garden" by the almanac.

4. Prepare a memory box of items that holds the special memories your loved one still relates to. This box can be used to redirect your loved one when they exhibit symptoms that are hard to manage. Appropriate items may include old photos of people who were most important in their life, particularly from their early adult period; tools or items used in their work environment; items that you can find at the thrift store that were used in the period when they were a young adult, etc. Remember that the best way for the caregiver to find R&R (rest and relaxation) is to provide R&R (redirection and reminiscing).

5. Include a variety of activities geared toward meeting physical, cognitive, and spiritual needs. Examples of activities that are often successful for persons living with Alzheimer's include picture recognition, coloring, Bible devotion, sing-a-longs, shape sorting,

memory box review, and old style games such as charades or Simon says. These types of activities are easy to execute and are often associated with one's long-term memory, and therefore are well received. They are also great opportunities for success.

6. Provide recreational activities that complement the individual's personal interests and hobbies. If someone enjoyed word puzzles, find easy level puzzles to solve. If someone enjoyed being outdoors, assist them to plant a container garden. If music was appreciated, provide the type of music they most enjoyed and sing along with them to their favorite song.

7. The key in regard to what type of activities to list will be to use the "meet me where I am" care approach. This requires some trial and error to find what they will respond to most readily and can accomplish successfully without being frustrated. Remember to provide opportunities for success throughout the day. It may be as simple as helping to fold washcloths, spreading peanut butter on the bread for sandwiches, or holding your hand. When tasks such as these are completed, it has a positive effect on self-esteem and individual motivation.

8. Inspect your home for hazards, including liquids, chemicals, medications, or other items that could be ingested, and make certain they are in secured areas out of your loved one's reach. A bottle of Clorox could resemble a gallon of milk to a patient with dementia. You can never be too safe! An additional concern is

to determine if exit-seeking activity is present. If so, continuous supervision will be required, or you may consider facility care to ensure safety.

9. Place written signs when needed to assist with verbal cuing to help your loved one find their way to places such as the bathroom. This can be particularly helpful when the patient begins urinating in inappropriate places, such as a closet that is mistakenly identified as an outhouse.

Remember that as the disease progresses, your loved one's needs will change. It is likely you will need to adjust the activities as time goes on in order to accommodate a successful outcome. DO NOT allow yourself to climb upon the "guilt train" if you find the burden of care is more than you can continue to provide in the home setting. Placing someone with Alzheimer's disease in a specialized program when they are no longer safe to live at home is an act of love, not abandonment.

We all have mentors in our life . . . someone who teaches us the ropes and takes us under their wings until we can fly on our own. For me, it was Ms. Eleanor. She was a nurse who inspired us all to give more, do better, and be proud of our profession. She was also the person who helped me learn not to take myself so seriously and to let go of the small stuff, something I was not very good at before meeting Ms. Eleanor. I was delighted years ago, when upon her retirement from the home health company we both worked for, to be the one who presented her with our parting gift: a pearl necklace to thank her for all the pearls of wisdom she had shared with us over the years.

Imagine my surprise when I saw her name listed as a new admission into one of the assisted living memory-care programs that I supported. Could it be my Ms. Eleanor was now a victim of Alzheimer's disease? I was hopeful that if it were her, she would remember me. In fact, I was sure she would. We had been very close once upon a time.

It did not take long to find out it was my dear, sweet Ms. Eleanor. She was near the end stages of the disease and had lost the ability to verbally communicate effectively as well as walk safely. When I first saw her, I barely recognized her. She was sitting in her wheelchair with a blank expression, staring off into space, oblivious to the world around her. I bent down beside her and told her who I was. She nodded her head slightly in acknowledgement, but there was no sign of recognition in her eyes. I was not fortunate enough to have known her in her younger days and it was hard for me to acknowledge that I was among the forgotten in her life.

I wanted so much to walk down memory lane with my old friend and talk about the good old days, the office pranks and the dreams she inspired within me. Yet I knew the only way to reach Ms. Eleanor was to go deeper into her memories to a time prior to my existence in her life. Taking her hand in mine, I began to talk to her of what I knew of her life, focusing on her husband whom she bragged about to all of us, her children, and her early career as a mental health nurse. While sharing stories I had heard about her yesterdays I could see a light of recognition growing in her eyes. She began to show interest and her focus changed from gazing into space to looking directly at me, especially when

I mentioned the names of the coworkers she worked closely with for many years. At first she gave only occasional nods, but that soon gave way to emphatic short sentences such as "Yes!" and "We had fun!" Eventually I was able to see her wearing the beautiful smile that she was once famous for. Now she looked like Ms. Eleanor, and it felt so good to be able to visit with her and see her personality come through. Had I remained selfish and tried to bring out a memory that we had personally shared, I would not have been able to experience the Ms. Eleanor I knew and loved.

There are millions of people throughout the world who carry the emotionally heavy and physically challenging title of Alzheimer's caregiver. It is a difficult journey to navigate, filled with many rocks and detours along the way. The paths must be chosen carefully, as we know the impact of our choices can make the difference between success and failure on any given day. Celebrate the good days. Comfort one another on the bad days. And continuously seek to "meet me where I am" while you enjoy your loved one to the fullest extent possible, helping them to reach their full potential with each day that passes.

Together, we *can* make a difference as we learn, understand, and give the best of our best while caring for those we know and love living with Alzheimer's disease.

*Those who hope in the Lord will renew their
strength. They will soar on wings like eagles;
they will run and not grow weary, they will
walk and not be faint.*

—Isaiah 40:31

Chapter Seven

# Quick-Start Questions and Answers

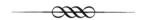

As a caregiver for a person living with Alzheimer's disease or a similar dementia, you have likely come to appreciate the precious value of time. Rarely does one wearing the title of caregiver report feeling they have time enough for any one thing, seeking knowledge included.

In speaking at dementia-care conferences, symposiums, and other settings from coast to coast, I have had the pleasure of meeting caregivers from all walks of life. Many seek answers to similar questions. This chapter is a compilation of the top twenty concerns brought to me by caregivers over the years. While there are sections throughout *Meet Me Where I Am* that touch on many of these topics, sometimes it is helpful to have key components of information readily available when you need it most. It is my hope this quick reference section will provide answers to some of your questions in a timely manner, thus giving back a little extra time for you to use where you need it most.

## What is the difference between Alzheimer's disease and dementia?

Imagine a giant umbrella with many raindrops of various sizes underneath. Have the image? Now, write the word *dementia* on the umbrella. The largest raindrop under the umbrella is Alzheimer's disease. The other raindrops represent the many other types of dementias that exist. Dementia is a general term used to describe a wide range of symptoms. Alzheimer's disease is a specific type of dementia accounting for 60 to 80 percent of all dementias. To have a diagnosis of dementia, one must have a decline in mental ability severe enough to interfere with daily life. Therefore, the primary difference between Alzheimer's disease and dementia is that dementia is a general term describing a set of symptoms, and Alzheimer's disease is a specific type of dementia.

## What causes Alzheimer's disease?

Alzheimer's is a neurodegenerative disease of the brain wherein brain cells die from protein abnormalities in the neuron. Over the course of time, tiny microscopic plaques (beta-amyloid proteins) and tangles (tau proteins) build up between and within the neurons of the brain, causing the cells to die. As the neurons die, there is a progressive loss of brain function that leads to the symptoms we know to be Alzheimer's disease. The first symptom recognized by most is a loss of short-term memory. The loss of brain function continues as neurons die until the brain itself ceases to function.

## What are the symptoms of Alzheimer's disease?

Everyone experiences moments when we can't think of a word we want to say, we forget an important date, or we walk into a room only to find ourselves retracing the reason we entered the room in the first place. When these moments occur more frequently than usual, we may wonder if something is wrong.

Think of it this way: it's not losing the car keys that should bother us, but rather finding them and not knowing what to do with them. Sometimes we stress over minor, everyday moments of forgetfulness that have nothing to do with the signs or symptoms of dementia. If you are concerned that you or a loved one is experiencing potential symptoms of dementia, it is always best to talk about these changes with a physician, for two reasons:

1. It never hurts to have a baseline cognitive test performed for future reference. If everyone had baseline testing when their brain was healthy, it would make detection of future changes easier should a dementia surface.

2. A physician can best determine if the concerns you have are normal experiences or if further testing is warranted.

The Alzheimer's Association has prepared a checklist to help identify the warning signs of dementia and includes guidance on what would be normal, age-related occurrences. This checklist is an excellent tool to use when preparing for a doctor's visit when symptoms of dementia are suspected. For your convenience, a copy of this checklist is shared on the following pages as found in the Alzheimer's Association website (www.alz.org).

## 10 SIGNS
### EARLY DETECTION MATTERS

# HAVE YOU NOTICED ANY OF THESE WARNING SIGNS?

Please list any concerns you have and take this sheet with you to the doctor.
*Note: This list is for information only and not a substitute for a consultation with a qualified professional.*

☐ 1. **MEMORY LOSS THAT DISRUPTS DAILY LIFE.** One of the most common signs of Alzheimer's disease, especially in the early stage, is forgetting recently learned information. Others include forgetting important dates or events, asking for the same information over and over, and increasingly needing to rely on aides (e.g., reminder notes or electronic devices) or family members for things they used to handle on their own. What's a typical age-related change? Sometimes forgetting names or appointments, but remembering them later.

_____

_____

☐ 2. **CHALLENGES IN PLANNING OR SOLVING PROBLEMS.** Some people may experience changes in their ability to develop and follow a plan or work with numbers. They may have trouble following a familiar recipe or keeping track of monthly bills. They may have difficulty concentrating and take much longer to do things than they did before. What's a typical age-related change? Making occasional errors when balancing a checkbook.

_____

_____

☐ 3. **DIFFICULTY COMPLETING FAMILIAR TASKS AT HOME, AT WORK OR AT LEISURE.** People with Alzheimer's disease often find it hard to complete daily tasks. Sometimes they may have trouble driving to a familiar location, managing a budget at work or remembering the rules of a favorite game. What's a typical age-related change? Occasionally needing help to use the settings on a microwave or to record a television show.

_____

_____

☐ 4. **CONFUSION WITH TIME OR PLACE.** People with Alzheimer's can lose track of dates, seasons and the passage of time. They may have trouble understanding something if it is not happening immediately. Sometimes they may forget where they are or how they got there. What's a typical age-related change? Getting confused about the day of the week but figuring it out later.

_____

_____

☐ 5. **TROUBLE UNDERSTANDING VISUAL IMAGES AND SPATIAL RELATIONSHIPS.** For some people, having vision problems is a sign of Alzheimer's. They may have difficulty reading, judging distance, and determining color or contrast, which may cause problems with driving. What's a typical age-related change? Vision changes related to cataracts.

_____

_____

☐ 6. **NEW PROBLEMS WITH WORDS IN SPEAKING OR WRITING.** People with Alzheimer's disease may have trouble following or joining a conversation. They may stop in the middle of a conversation and have no idea how to continue or they may repeat themselves. They may struggle with vocabulary, have problems finding the right word or call things by the wrong name (e.g., calling a "watch" a "hand clock").
What's a typical age-related change? Sometimes having trouble finding the right word.

☐ 7. **MISPLACING THINGS AND LOSING THE ABILITY TO RETRACE STEPS.** A person with Alzheimer's may put things in unusual places. They may lose things and be unable to go back over their steps to find them again. Sometimes, they may accuse others of stealing. This may occur more frequently over time.
What's a typical age-related change? Misplacing things from time to time and retracing steps to find them.

☐ 8. **DECREASED OR POOR JUDGMENT.** People with Alzheimer's may experience changes in judgment or decision making. For example, they may use poor judgment when dealing with money, giving large amounts to telemarketers. They may pay less attention to grooming or keeping themselves clean.
What's a typical age-related change? Making a bad decision once in a while.

☐ 9. **WITHDRAWAL FROM WORK OR SOCIAL ACTIVITIES.** A person with Alzheimer's disease may start to remove themselves from hobbies, social activities, work projects or sports. They may have trouble keeping up with a favorite sports team or remembering how to complete a favorite hobby. They may also avoid being social because of the changes they have experienced.
What's a typical age-related change? Sometimes feeling weary of work, family and social obligations.

☐ 10. **CHANGES IN MOOD AND PERSONALITY.** The mood and personalities of people with Alzheimer's can change. They can become confused, suspicious, depressed, fearful or anxious. They may be easily upset at home, at work, with friends or in places where they are out of their comfort zone.
What's a typical age-related change? Developing very specific ways of doing things and becoming irritable when a routine is disrupted.

If you or someone you care about is experiencing any of the 10 Warning Signs of Alzheimer's disease, please see a doctor to find the cause. Early diagnosis gives you a chance to seek treatment and plan for your future.
The Alzheimer's Association can help. Visit **alz.org/10signs** or call **800.272.3900** (TTY: 866.403.3073).

## Is Alzheimer's disease hereditary?

When we have family members diagnosed with Alzheimer's disease it is natural to worry whether our personal risks of being diagnosed in the future are increased.
Research indicates when we have *immediate* family members with Alzheimer's, such as a parent or sibling, we are
at a higher risk. If we have more than one close family
member diagnosed, the risks are increased. It is not always
clear in such circumstances how much is due to genetics
and how much is due to environmental factors. Yet the truth
is, regardless of family history, everyone is at risk for developing Alzheimer's disease. The greatest risk factor for this
disease is aging. One in three persons in America over the
age of eighty has Alzheimer's, regardless of family history.

While genetic components do exist, it is still unclear
how to interpret what all of the data means when determining one's specific risks. For example, there are certain *risk
genes* that have been identified with the development of
Alzheimer's disease. Just because you carry the risk gene
does not mean you will definitely experience Alzheimer's
disease. The apolipoprotein E-e4, or APOE-e4, was the first
risk gene identified. A second category of genes known as
*deterministic genes* are rare, accounting for less than 1 percent of all cases. A person who carries a deterministic gene
*will* develop Alzheimer's disease, usually showing symptoms by their fourth or fifth decade of life. In these rare
families, the history of Alzheimer's disease is extremely
high. Many of these families are being followed in research
studies. It is hoped by studying those carrying a deterministic gene science will be able to find a cure.

If someone is very concerned about their genetic risks, they may consider seeking the guidance of a genetic counselor. While genetic testing is now available to determine if you carry a risk gene, remember, this does not mean you *will* develop Alzheimer's disease. The Alzheimer's Association, as well as experts in general, do not recommend genetic testing unless you are advised to do so by a genetic counselor. If you believe your family history warrants further personal evaluation, and would like to access a genetic counselor, you can find more information at the National Society of Genetic Counselors website (www.nsgc.org).

## Can Alzheimer's disease be prevented?

To date there is no proven way to prevent Alzheimer's disease. Research continues to work on breaking the code to understand what causes the protein abnormalities in the neurons of the Alzheimer's brain in hopes of finding a cure. Until this breakthrough is found, there are measures we can take to decrease our individual risk factors. The number one risk factor for developing Alzheimer's disease is aging, something we all want to do! While we age, we must do all we can to take great care of our brain. An organ that is weak is more likely to succumb to illness. The brain is the master organ of the body. When we focus on maintaining our brain at the healthiest, most functional level possible, we are actually decreasing our chances of being diagnosed with diseases such as Alzheimer's. Below you will find an easy way to practice healthy brain habits and thus reduce any personal risk factors:

**T** = Take time for you! Rest when needed. Sleep seven to eight hours each night.

**H** = Have a healthy daily diet, such as the Mediterranean diet.

**I** = Improve your mental health, especially if you feel depressed or blue.

**N** = Needing others and staying social is important in all stages of life, especially as you age.

**K** = Kick bad habits! Smoking decreases blood flow to the brain and other organs.

**H** = "Helmet hair is beautiful" is a quote to remember. Brain injuries increase your risks.

**E** = Engage as often as possible in cognitively stimulating activities.

**A** = Aspire to exercise routinely. Don't be a couch potato!

**L** = Live a "heart healthy" lifestyle. If it's good for your heart, it's good for your brain.

**T** = Tranquility is good for you! Try to keep your stress to a minimum.

**H** = Higher education can be fun, but especially good for the brain as you age.

## Is there a test to detect Alzheimer's disease?

There is no single test to definitively diagnosis Alzheimer's disease on a living person. After one has passed away, some families request an autopsy to verify the diagnosis. In most cases due to the guidelines clinicians must follow to make such a diagnosis, the autopsy validates the diagnosis to be correct, though not always. To diagnose Alzheimer's disease, the first step is to review what is experienced by the individual and/or reported by the caregiver. Once the history is reviewed, the physician will perform a complete physical examination and a battery of tests, including cognitive and psychological screenings, brain imaging, and blood laboratory studies, to name a few. The goal of the physician will be to determine any and all sources that could be causing the dementia symptoms. Once all the data is in and test results reviewed, the medical team can make a confident diagnosis. In certain cases, there will be clinical information to support the diagnosis, such as a brain image that indicates Alzheimer's disease is likely.

## How important is it to seek a specific dementia diagnosis?

Dementia by itself is not a specific disease, but rather a general term used to describe a group of symptoms involving memory loss, reasoning ability, and social skills to the extent they interfere with daily functioning. There are many specific diseases that cause dementia, such as Alzheimer's disease, vascular dementia, Lewy body dementia, and frontotemporal dementia, to name a few. In some cases, it is found a person may experience more than one type of dementia. When dementia symptoms are first identified, the physician will usually work to seek the exact cause of the symptoms for several reasons:

1.  Knowing the specific cause (type) of the dementia helps to determine what to expect as the disease progresses.

2.  While most dementias are progressive and irreversible, certain types may be halted or reversed with treatment, such as normal pressure hydrocephalus.

3.  When physicians seek to identify the specific cause of the dementia symptoms, it is sometimes identified as a nondementia medical issue, such as a brain tumor, endocrine dysfunction, dehydration, or encephalopathy, to name a few.

**What are the stages of Alzheimer's disease?**

This can be a confusing question as it depends on what reference you use. A commonly recognized scale developed by Dr. Barry Reisberg of New York University defines seven stages, beginning with no impairment and ending with very severe decline. The Mayo Clinic defines five stages, beginning with preclinical Alzheimer's disease and ending with severe Alzheimer's disease. Each scale is consistent in that the disease begins long before the first symptoms appear. It is now believed that changes in the Alzheimer's brain may begin as early as twenty years before the first symptoms surface. Once diagnosed, the average life span is between four and eight years, though some have lived as long as twenty years, and others will progress rapidly to end stages within a year or two of being diagnosed. The Alzheimer's Association simplifies the explanation of Alzheimer's staging, describing three basic stages: mild (early stage), moderate (middle stage), and severe (late stage). The Alzheimer's Association calls the period of time prior to any symptoms manifesting, the "preclinical" period of Alzheimer's disease. For ease of understanding, we will use the model discussed in the Alzheimer's Association website (www.alz.org) to explain the stages of Alzheimer's disease.

In the early stage, a person is usually aware of issues, such as not being to recall the names of new people they meet, difficulty finding the right words in conversations, and some challenges with problem solving. Certain individuals have been known to still drive or even stay employed during the early stages.

In the middle stage, symptoms progress to include confusion to place and setting, wandering of the exit-seeking type, issues related to paranoias, and difficulty recognizing close family members. The person may become resistant to care, have issues with bowel and bladder continence, and will demonstrate a general decline in their ability to meet their own hygiene needs.

In the late stage, one will progressively decline, losing the ability to walk, communicate, and even feed themselves. Weight loss is typical in this stage, even when someone feeds them, as their body becomes unable to process the nutrients received. They will become dependent on their caregiver to meet all of their care needs, including toileting, bathing, dressing, grooming, and mobility. There is a high risk of respiratory infections such as pneumonia in the late stage, and often this is the cause of death.

## How can I convince someone to go the doctor if I suspect there is an issue, but they refuse to go?

Sometimes the person who is exhibiting symptoms of dementia is resistant to the thought of going to a physician for medical evaluation. There are many reasons one might refuse to go. One could be afraid of what the assessment might reveal. Another is denial that a problem exists. Convincing a person to seek medical attention who does not wish to do so is a difficult task, but you must try your best when the symptoms of dementia are present to determine the cause and subsequent treatment. The following are a few suggestions that might be helpful:

- Ask the person if they have noticed any changes in their memory, in problem solving, or in other areas of managing their daily life. It is always best if you can get them to first identify any problems that may exist. If they can see the problem, they may be more likely to agree to go for a medical evaluation.

- Try talking openly with the person, sharing what you have observed and why it is important for them to see a doctor. Explain that because you care about them and want to make sure there is nothing wrong with their heart, their blood vessels, their brain, or any other part of their body, you would like to go with them to the doctor to talk about the changes you are seeing.

- Assure them they will have the opportunity to personally talk with the doctor about their feelings and any symptoms they believe to be present or if they disagree with what you personally have brought to their attention.

- Be sure to address any concerns or fears they have, reassuring them you will be there with them.

- Be prepared for a possible emotional reaction if they are in denial of their symptoms or if fear of admitting something is wrong is driving their refusal to see the physician.

If all efforts have failed, and you hold a health-care power of attorney with the required HIPPA authorizations to do so, reapproach by attempting to set up an appointment for an "annual physical," making certain you communicate your concerns with the physician in advance of the visit. A routine visit with a physician they know and trust is not seen as a negative event. This can be a useful approach for individuals who are adamant that "nothing is wrong" and are less than cooperative in working with you to arrange an assessment.

In some areas, you may find there are physicians who make house calls. If the dementia symptoms are so prevalent that paranoias are present and the person refuses to leave their home, this may be a helpful resource. You can research such options online and discuss the situation in advance with the visiting practice. A helpful approach I have seen in such situations is for the visiting physician to meet your loved one over a cup of coffee to get the conversation started. During the visit, introduce your new friend who happens to be a doctor. You may find your loved one is willing to openly discuss their health in the comfort of their home with the new family friend who happens to be a doctor.

## How can I find information on support groups in my area?

Support groups come in all shapes and sizes, meet in many settings, and can be an important path in the caregiving journey. Finding the right support group for you can be a difficult task. Caregiving is often a full-time job. It is not always easy to find the time necessary to research the support groups that are available in your area. Your local chapter of the Alzheimer's Association keeps a listing of active support groups and can provide information in regard to the general makeup of each group. Are you looking for one just for spouses? A group that is small and intimate? Or is the location more important to you? There are also a number of online support groups that are growing in popularity. The internet is a great resource for this type of forum. Simply type "Alzheimer's support groups online" and you will find many options to explore.

## Where can I find assistance with the burden of caregiving costs?

According to statistics published by the Alzheimer's Association, the costs of persons living with dementia totaled $259 billion for 2017. Medicare and Medicaid paid approximately half of these expenses, leaving the rest to be paid by funds such as insurance, retirement plans, life savings, and family members. This does not take into account the estimated 18.2 billion unpaid caregiver hours provided by family, friends, and volunteers and valued at another $230 billion. Knowing where to look to ensure you are accessing all the benefits and funds available in chronic illness scenarios is important for all involved. Your local Council on Aging office may be aware of community-based programs with special grants or waiver programs that could be of help. If the patient or their spouse ever served in the military, there may be benefits available through the Veterans Administration that are specific to dementia care expenses. In addition, consider visiting the websites below for additional information regarding benefits, resources, and payment options for care needs:

Benefits Check Up, National Council on Aging,
www.benefitscheckup.org

Benefits.gov,
www.benefits.gov

Centers for Medicare & Medicaid Services,
www.cms.gov

US Department of Social Security,
www.ssa.gov/medicare/prescriptionhelp/

The SHIP National Technical Assistance Center,
www.shiptacenter.org

Partnership for Prescription Assistance, www.pparx.org

**How do I practice "meet me where I am" care when it feels like a lie to do so?**

Occasionally someone will tell me at times they feel like they are telling a lie to their loved one when trying "meet me where I am" care and are compelled to correct their loved ones or tell the truth of a situation. For example, a wife asks when her husband will be home. Her husband actually passed away years ago. In this example, I would advise the caregiver that it would be wrong to tell the wife—who believes her husband is alive—he passed away years ago. We have to understand in the "meet me where I am" care philosophy the wife requires the caregiver to journey with her into her past, a time when her husband was very much alive. This place and time in truth existed for this wife and was not a lie, but rather a beautiful thread from the tapestry of her past that her broken brain clings to.

Alzheimer's disease tosses memories around without respect to accuracy of place and time. Acknowledging the reality of one's memories is not only truth, it is also medicine to their well-being. This wife has no control over how her memories flow from moment to moment. To uproot her from a pleasant past where her husband lives beside her, only to abruptly bring her to a reality where he ceases to exist, would create a flood of sudden sadness, not to mention probable denial and increased confusion as her broken memories tell her otherwise. Thus, it is not a lie to enter the truth that is presented from one's past.

It is true we cannot produce the husband she seeks, thus in this example, telling the wife her husband will be home soon may not be the best answer. What can we do then that acknowledges her moment, gains her trust, and prevents the need to bring tragic news into an otherwise pleasant reality? Simply say something that would be appropriate for her memory's timeline—something that she can accept—then quickly redirect her attention to something of interest that engages her otherwise. One response that would be appropriate would be: "Dad can't be here right now, but while we are here together, let's make some of his favorite cookies!" Or maybe you start a sing-along or some other activity that you know the person will enjoy. The key in such situations is to first acknowledge the focus in a way that provides a sense of calm and comfort, then do your best to redirect and engage the person in an activity that helps their short-term memory reset.

## How do I know when to take over the tasks of daily care?

Each day it is likely you bathe and dress yourself. While we don't think of these simple daily tasks in such terms, getting ready for the day is a personal success. Now imagine you are suddenly no longer able to care for yourself. You are completely dependent on another person to do your entire morning routine, including putting on your deodorant, brushing your teeth, and even buttoning your clothing. How does it feel? For most of us the thought is unsettling, to say the least.

When providing care for persons living with dementia in early and middle stages, the goals are, as always, to allow the person to do as much for themselves as possible. Completion of the task is far more important than perfection. We become used to the mismatched sock, the striped pants paired with a flowered shirt, and other wardrobe abnormalities as we practice "meet me where I am" care. Our barometer is the person's affect. Are they happy with their appearance, regardless of your personal perceptions or judgments? Are they participating with their care? Does the person show interest in their grooming? As long as the person is actively participating, showing interest, and happy with their appearance, you have a success!

This does not mean you won't have to intervene and assist in areas where they are not able to fully meet their own needs. Often there will be a tag team of care where you allow the individual to do a much for themselves as they can, while you complete the hygiene they are not able to do on their own. For example, a mother in the middle stage of Alzheimer's dressed herself every day. The problem was she became fixated on one particular outfit and was putting dirty clothes on each day. The daughter became creative and bought five identical pink polo shirts with matching mint-green jeans. She collected the dirty clothes each night, laying the clean ones out each morning. Problem solved!

As the dementia progresses, you will notice the desire to dress and groom oneself begins to diminish. Personal hygiene becomes poor. They no longer brush their own hair. They show no interest in what they wear or even attempt to change their own clothing. These are signals that the disease has progressed and the person is now completely dependent on the caregiver for all grooming and hygiene tasks. It is good to ease into the process with attempts to invite their participation using simple yes or no questions to determine whether there is any desire left to participate in their own care. For example, let's say it is time to dress for the day. You may enlist the person's participation by asking if they would like to wear the yellow dress or the green dress. Next, when it is time to put on shoes, offer a choice between two pairs of shoes. This allows for individual involvement and input at a lower level while transitioning to full care status.

## How do I know when something is medically wrong when Alzheimer's disease complicates effective communication?

Parents of young children recognize when their children are less active or have a sleepless night, which often cues the parent to examine their health. Irritable day? Grab the thermometer to check for a fever or the flashlight for a red throat. Even if there are no obvious signs of illness, if a young child isn't eating or playing like they normally do, we are usually quick to take them to see the doctor. We celebrate when children reach the age they can tell us when they are not feeling well.

When dementia is present, caregivers may find themselves having similar feelings while trying to recognize when an illness is present and whether it is time to schedule a doctor's visit. Persons living with dementia often do not complain when they feel physically ill. Some are no longer capable of verbal communication. Others may feel certain symptoms, yet the damaged cells in their brain prevent effective communication of what they are experiencing. If the person you are caring for has reached a stage where they can no longer communicate when they are feeling bad, they will likely show you in other ways. Look for a sudden decline in eating, sleeping, toileting or other abilities, or a sudden withdrawal or disinterest in their usual routine. Another sign illness may be present would be a sudden increase in agitation or aggression with no apparent reason. When such events occur, it is a good practice to seek a medical evaluation to rule out illness as the potential cause.

## What should I worry about in regard to safety concerns?

Diseases that damage brain cells affect one's ability to think clearly, problem solve appropriately, and make rational decisions. Because of this, there are multiple components involved in maintaining a safe environment for persons living with dementias. The following lists some of the more critical measures to consider in order to keep your loved one safe. Remember, these recommendations are not a replacement for personal supervision of individuals who are no longer safe when at home or living alone.

### Location Safety

When Alzheimer's or other dementias are diagnosed, consider the use of a GPS tracking watch, bracelet, or another wearable device. While an individual may still be able to correctly identify their physical location as well as where they want to go, remember that Alzheimer's and similar dementias are progressive. Eventually there will come a time when they will not know where they are and may try to leave their current location to seek a place that is more familiar. This is an emergency situation. There are far too many cases of people who became lost in their own neighborhoods when they left the safety and security of their own homes to find the *home* they remembered. In some cases, people were safely returned by neighbors or others who knew them. In other cases, the outcome was not so good, including loss of life for persons who wandered into rural settings and were not found in time. There are many programs that specialize in safe return devices that link to smartphone apps or other easy to use technology that help unite loved ones when needed.

Sundowning is a common phenomenon that occurs when the caregiver says "goodnight" and the person living with dementia finds the need to get up for various reasons. Day can become night and night can become day when dementia is present. While you are sleeping soundly, your loved one may get up at two in the morning to ready themselves for work, try to cook a meal, or quietly wander and plunder about the house. Baby monitors and dead bolts are not an appropriate substitute for supervision of the person who has begun to sundown during the sleeping hours of the caregiver. When this symptom manifests, it is time for 24/7 care to ensure safety. Options to consider include hiring caregivers to assist you in the home setting, as no one individual could or should attempt to try 24/7 care, or seeking placement in one of the many special-care program communities designed especially for persons living with dementia.

## Driving Safety

We must be respectful of the fact that just because a person has dementia does not automatically mean they are not capable of safe driving. Likewise, just because a person refuses to give up the car keys when they are no longer driving safely doesn't mean they should continue to drive. While most individuals living with dementia independently choose to surrender their car keys for safety purposes once diagnosed, some individuals exercise their right to drive for as long as possible. If the person living with dementia is still driving, be sure to assess their driving ability frequently to determine safety and ability. Knowing what to look for and how to address issues when they arrive is important. Are response times to stop signs and traffic signals appropriate?

Are they hesitating at intersections or other points requiring decisions? Are there issues in finding their way from one point to another? Have there been any traffic incidents?

When issues such as these begin to occur, it is best to seek a driving evaluation by the physician. It is likely the physician will determine they are no longer safe to drive and ask that they surrender their license. In such situations, it is important to have open and honest conversations, acknowledging the person's feelings while explaining the observations as to why driving is no longer safe. If they refuse to cease driving, solicit the assistance of a trusted authority, such as a police officer who observed erratic driving, or take them to the department of motor vehicles for a driving test. You can also ask other family members to talk about the risks of harm not only to themselves but also to others, should the person living with dementia continue to drive.

## Environment Safety

One of the greatest risks of injury for persons living with dementia is the risk of injury from ingestion. Keep any and all medications, chemicals, laundry products, fluids, powders, or other items that could be consumed, drunk, or otherwise ingested safely stored and away from access. Also consider other hazards for injury in settings such as kitchens, garages, and workshops. Sharp objects, machinery, and even hot water can pose serious threats when judgment is impaired. Remove and/or disable machinery that would be injurious if operated inappropriately. Stoves and ovens are also hazards when left unsupervised. Many electrical devices can be placed on keyed systems with the assistance of an electrician. You may consider this option for safety purposes. It is also recommended to locate door locks higher or lower than usual for persons who are prone to unlocking exit doors.

## Physical Safety

As dementias progress, risks for falls will increase. Keep the walking environment well-lit and free of throw rugs. Smooth, one-level surfaces are best. Have the person cared for wear shoes that are well fitted and low to the ground and try to avoid shoe laces that may become untied. Daily exercise helps to maintain muscle tone, which in turn can help prevent falls. Supervise bath and shower time to prevent falls, and install grab bars in the bathroom where needed. Walk-in showers are safer and more convenient than tubs that require one to take a large step over the side. If the person shows signs of tiring during the shower routine, use a shower chair or stool to prevent falling. Place nonslip surfaces in the bottom of tubs and showers.

Be prepared for emergencies, as you will have little time to collect needed information when emergencies occur. Have a list prepared in advance with all medical information, including a complete medical history, all medications prescribed including doses and times, the names and phone numbers of all physicians, and any allergies. This list should go with your loved one any time they go to a doctor, emergency room, or hospital. You should also keep a complete listing of all emergency numbers you might have cause to access should the need arise, such as the poison control hotline or medical or fire department phone numbers outside of 911 in your area.

Last but not least, at all times keep an emergency "safe return" kit to be used by officials in the event your loved one ever becomes lost. In this kit you should have a current photo of your loved one, a piece of clothing worn by your loved one that would have their scent on it sealed in a plastic bag to be used by police dogs, a list of any addresses your loved one might remember that could be places they would seek as "home" or familiar locations.

**How is music used to stimulate memories?**

Using music as therapy can be a very beneficial activity for individuals living with Alzheimer's and other dementias when performed correctly. The key is knowing what specific music was enjoyed by the person living with dementia during their late teens and into their early thirties. Was there a special song associated with a magic moment in life? A tune that, no matter what, brought a smile to their face? These are the songs that can bring magic moments to life and restore memories once believed to be forgotten.

Research has proven that music stimulates a part of the brain in the limbic system known as the hippocampus, which plays a special role in the storage of memories. I have had the pleasure of witnessing many times how memories once believed to be forgotten can suddenly be restored when specific music is presented. One of my favorite observations was when a lady in advanced stages of Alzheimer's was first given a playlist of songs on an MP3 player using a set of headphones. This sweet woman could no longer walk, had lost the ability to use intelligible speech, and seemingly no longer recognized her husband, who was present when the earphones were first placed on her head. His comment prior to the experiment was, "I don't think this will do much good since she doesn't notice much of anything anymore." The first song she heard was the tune that played when she and her husband danced on their wedding day. Her husband had provided several selections of songs he thought might be of interest that he knew she used to be fond of.

When we first placed the headphones over her ears and turned on the music, we were disappointed that there was no response. Her flat affect and blank stare continued. Then halfway through the first chorus of "Fly Me to the Moon" we watched in awe as her eyes opened a little wider and she looked more closely at the man standing in front of her. She began to reach for him. He walked closer to her. When he stood within her reach, she grabbed hold of his shirt, using what little strength she had to pull herself to a standing position from her wheelchair. Suddenly she began to smile as she laid her head on his shoulder and softly swayed to the memories of yesteryear. Her husband held her in his arms with tears rolling down his cheeks in disbelief. His wife had been lost to him for so long, but now here she was, his bride, swaying to their song! This is the magic of music and memory—combining the special songs of yesterday so that memories can find their way into today.

## How do you talk to children about Alzheimer's disease?

The Alzheimer's family has many members who are affected when a loved one is diagnosed, including children. In recent years a number of books have been written explaining dementia to young children, including one that I coau-thored with Dr. Beatrice Tauber Prior, titled *Grandma and Me: A Kid's Guide for Alzheimer's and Dementia*. Books are a great way to provide gentle, age-appropriate informa-tion to start the necessary conversations with children about Alzheimer's disease and what they can expect when a loved one is diagnosed. Children have greater insight than they are sometimes given credit for. We should encourage children to ask questions, to talk about their feelings and their fears.

Trying to separate children from Alzheimer's loved ones to protect them from potential negative interactions is not the best solution. Rather, it is recommended to educate the child, explaining what is going on in their loved one's brain, and to promote pleasant visits and interactions between the child and the person living with dementia. There may be times when it is appropriate to remove the child from the care setting. Such times would include when difficult symptoms manifest, like anxiety, paranoia, or anger. Oth-erwise, be supportive of interactions between the child and the person living with dementia and allow interactions to naturally occur in a supervised setting. Continue to provide support as long as the child is comfortable.

A child may be afraid they have done something wrong, which has caused their loved one to treat them differently than before. Once they understand that their loved one has an illness that is causing the changes, they are more likely to lose their fears and accept the changes. One analogy chil-dren seem to understand is to explain that Alzheimer's dis-ease is like having a broken arm. With Alzheimer's, the part of the body that is broken is in the brain—the brain doesn't work like it did before it was broken. Because of the broken part of the brain, their loved one has problems with how they remember things, how they think, and how they sometimes act. Let the child know they can't catch Alzheimer's disease like they can catch a cold, so there is no reason to be afraid to be around their loved one. The broken part of the brain will cause their grandma, grandpa, or loved one to sometimes say things or do things they do not usually say or do. Explaining that sometimes people who have Alzheimer's show they are sick by being sad or mad is helpful so that when these moments occur, children understand it is the Alzheimer's disease and not the person causing the moment.

## How do I take the battle out of the bathing?

Consider the bathroom of your dreams. What do you imagine? Is it a glass shower with granite walls, multiple showerheads, and a wide bench seat to rest upon? Maybe you are a romantic at heart, and your first thoughts were of a deep, white tub surrounded by candles, overflowing with bubbles, with the smell of lavender and soft music in the background.

Whatever your vision, it likely you had little trouble thinking of what you would create if you could. It is also likely your mental creation had little resemblance to the tiny bathrooms with the crocheted toilet-paper holders and matching furry lid covers representing the bathrooms of yesteryear. For one in advancing stages of Alzheimer's, entering a modern bathroom might feel like they are entering a spaceship. Even today's modern commodes have little resemblance to the older style toilets used long ago.

In the battle of the bathroom, one challenge is the design of modern bathrooms has changed so much that persons living with dementia sometimes fail to understand that entering the bathroom environment represents a need for a shower or the need for toileting. A second challenge can be how invasive and intimate it feels to have clothing taken off, regardless of the reason. When a person with Alzheimer's fails to completely recognize the reasoning why they must remove their clothing, their natural inclination is to resist and to fight. These are just a few of the many reasons caregivers experience battles in the bathroom in dementia care settings.

To decrease the battles in the bathroom and increase opportunities for success, caregivers need to use auditory, visual, and tactile cuing prior to bathing and toileting experiences. For example, show the Alzheimer's patient a picture card with a nostalgic-looking bathroom in color and write the task you seek to accomplish in clear, large print at the top of the card. When it is time to take a bath, show the card with an image of the bath and the word "bath" written clearly across the top and state, "It is time to take a bath." Be sure to point to the bath picture. Give them the card and let them look at the picture for a moment or two while you gather the supplies. Have all the needed toiletries including soap, towel, and oral care items ready in an easy to grab tote. Upon reapproach, with an outstretched hand, a smile, and showing excitement, ask the person to follow you. If there is a particular toiletry the person always used with their bathing, such as a specific powder or certain brand of soap, place the toiletry under their nose so they can smell the aroma. The olfactory sense has long-term connection with memory. The aroma of a scent that is commonly associated with the task can also help to persuade one's mind that it is time to perform the task.

Be sure to have the water flowing and heated appropriately prior to entering the bathroom, placing all necessary supplies within reach. Try including the person with dementia as much as possible in the process rather than just bathing them. The ability to mimic is one of the last skill sets we lose, so showing and demonstrating motions on yourself may be helpful. There is an old technique called "see one, do one, teach one" that can be a helpful process. For example, soap the washcloth, explaining you are getting the washcloth ready for the bath. This would be the "show one" step. Rub the washcloth up and down on your arm and comment on how nice the soap feels. This is the "do one" step. Now hand the washcloth to the person with Alzheimer's and ask them to wash their own arms. This would cover the component "teach one." Your goal is always to decrease the fears, anxieties, and paranoias often associated with bathing and dementia, thus subsequently decreasing the battles. You may find you have to try multiple approaches before identifying the one(s) that work best for you and the person you care for. When all else fails, try giving a sponge bath.

**What is the right way to approach the person living with dementia and how should I communicate?**

Have you ever been in a crowded room, lost in your own thoughts, when someone touched you on the shoulder from behind to get your attention? When this happens to me, I'm like a cat from a cartoon, jumping for the ceiling. I feel the blood rush through my body as my autonomic nervous system speeds up my heart and prepares me for the fight or flight response. Luckily in the split seconds that follow, I turn to recognize a familiar face. My heart rate slows and I relax because my brain is able to quickly ascertain I am safe. When such moments occur for people living with Alzheimer's disease, the outcome can be quite different. The damaged brain cells do not always send the "all clear" message when they are abruptly approached or startled, causing the autonomic system that was initially activated to stay in full gear. Rather than calming down when the source of the interruption is identified, responses are escalated and may include defensive maneuvers such as pulling away, yelling, running, or even becoming combative. In order to avoid creating a negative response, consider the following tips when approaching individuals living with Alzheimer's disease and other dementias:

1. Maintain a positive demeanor, wear a smile, and be sure to make eye contact as you approach.

2. Do not stand over a person who is sitting down. Pull a chair beside them or kneel so that you are on the same level.

3. Never approach someone from behind or from the side, but rather make your approach in the front of their visual field. As Alzheimer's progresses, peripheral vision tends to narrow and the focus of the visual field tends to shift downward.

4. Do not assume someone sees you just because you are standing in front of them. Call their name and

say hello, seeking eye contact to acknowledge they see you.

5. Before touching someone, stretch your hand out in their direction, palm up, as if you are reaching for their hand. This is a universal symbol that you are asking for their permission to make physical contact. Often you will receive an answer—the person will reach back and hold your hand. This is a certain sign that permission has been granted. If they do not automatically reach for your hand, and you feel the need to touch a person to console them, tell them what you are going to do in advance. For example: "I would like to give you hug if that is okay with you. I feel like I could use a hug too." As you maintain eye contact, keeping your positive smile, gently test the waters as you touch their arm. If there is no resistance you may proceed with the hug.

Communicating with Alzheimer's patients requires careful considerations to ensure optimal success. Never try to argue or use logic when making a point or trying to convince the Alzheimer's patient of your point of view. "Meet me where I am" care philosophy teaches us it is best to acknowledge the person with Alzheimer's perceptions and beliefs as their reality as a first step in all communication. Once we enter into their moment, we gain their trust. If the issue is a paranoia where the person is focused on money they believe to be stolen or a possession they believe to be missing, assure them the item they seek is safe, then do your best to redirect their attention to another topic, and offer reminiscence therapy to bring the person to a better place as you reset their short-term memory.

We process information three ways: auditory (what we hear), visual (what we see), and tactile (what we feel). We should attempt to present all communication in all three forms to increase the opportunity for successful reception when communicating with persons who have Alzheimer's disease. For example, you want to tell your husband it is time to eat. You have prepared one of his favorites for lunch, peanut butter and jelly sandwiches. The way to present this information using auditory, visual, and tactile communication would be to hold up a sandwich and say, "It is time for lunch. I have made your favorite! Peanut butter and jelly sandwiches!" As you tell him what you made, place half of a sandwich in his hand. You have now used all three forms of communication, telling him about the sandwich, showing it to him, and letting him physically hold it. The chances that your husband will now eat the sandwich has increased exponentially.

When asking questions, use simple sentences that present either-or options or call for yes or no responses in order to avoid overwhelming the person living with dementia. For example, "What would you like to do today?" can be met with a flat affect or even frustration from the person living with dementia since this question requires a lot of brain matter to process. A better approach would be something like, "Would you like to sit outside for a while?"

Try reading nonverbal cues as much as possible when communicating, being aware of your own body language at all times. Studies indicate only 30 percent of all communication is verbal. The remainder is dependent on components such as voice inflection, body language, affect, and other nonverbal cues. If your affect is nervous, anxious, or less than confident, this is what the person you are caring for will hear. Likewise, if the person cared for says they feel okay, but they are pacing, acting nervous, and fidgeting, it is likely they need you to respond to their actions, not their words, and help them find a better place within.

As dementias progress, the ability to speak intelligibly will decrease. Some people will lose all speech capabilities and become dependent on hand gestures. Knowing how to read body language in these stages is extremely important. Is there a particular part of the body they are no longer moving? Evaluate this area for potential injury. Is there a new or sudden activity manifesting that has never existed before? This could be some way of communicating a need or desire. A woman who wanted to go the bathroom had no way of asking for her needs to be met, but would go around patting people on the arm and smiling. With some trial and error, the staff caring for her eventually figured out this was her signal. A man who suddenly started kicking everyone that walked by was eventually diagnosed with a blood clot in his leg. Again, it was his body language that led to the identification of his problem.

Conversations are most successful when conducted in quiet environments with minimal distractions. Be patient and allow adequate time for the Alzheimer's patient to respond. Avoid talking for them or talking over them. It is typical for the person with dementia to have difficulty finding the right words, to become easily distracted, and to feel frustrated when they can't say what they are trying to express. Offering reassurance and being patient is necessary to facilitate effective communication.

## Why is meaningful, engaging activity so important in dementia care?

From the moment we take our first breath a timeline begins marking the moments of our lives. There are many events to celebrate. First words, first steps, first bike ride, first car, first kiss, and even first love. We continue adding to our timeline as we age, starting families and careers and doing what is expected of us. Education? Check. Providing for our family? Check. Taking care of ourselves? Well, at least we try. Time passes and the story of life unfolds, with each defining moment a golden thread in our tapestry.

But with dementia, the key to creating meaningful activities is to seek "opportunities for success." Too often we approach individuals who have dementia with a mindset of *disability*, thinking only of what the person can no longer do. While this is necessary to consider in daily care, it is also necessary to be mindful of the *ability* still present, doing our best to capitalize on what can still be done independently, even if it is not performed perfectly. As loving and willful caregivers we have a tendency to take over all tasks, leaving the dementia patient with nothing to do other than sit around and become bored. To be left without cognitive, physical, sensory, and spiritual stimulation will lead to restlessness, sleep disruption, inability to focus, and an increased potential for combative behaviors. Providing meaningful, enjoyable activities that are appropriate to one's individual skill set provides the stimulation needed, increases confidence, and helps everyone feel more successful at the end of the day.

The best type of activity depends on individual interests, abilities, and what stage of the disease process a person is in. For example, if someone always enjoyed completing crossword puzzles, they may enjoy simplified, large print puzzles deep into the middle stages of Alzheimer's disease. If a person never showed interest in word puzzles, it is unlikely this would be an enjoyable activity. In the advanced stages of Alzheimer's, once the ability to speak, walk, and feed one's self is lost, a successful activity could be giving someone a hand massage while looking into their eyes and telling them how much you appreciate their spending time with you.

Laughter is important too! Have fun whenever and however possible. Something as simple as playing balloon volleyball while sitting in chairs face to face is a great activity and good physical exercise. It may take a few attempts before you are comfortable conducting daily activities, but one thing is certain: the closer you come to an individual's long-term hobbies, likes, interests, and routine, the closer you will be to creating magic moments in your caregiving journey!

Here are some additional suggestions for creative activities:

### *Sing like no one is listening!*

No matter what the stage of disease process, singing a familiar tune out loud, such as "Jingle Bells," "You Are My Sunshine," or their favorite song, usually elicits a positive response. You may even find that individuals who no longer communicate verbally can still hum or follow along with you in a sing-along of familiar lyrics.

### Take a stroll down memory lane together.

As mentioned in previous sections, reminiscence therapy is a powerful tool that can be done any time two or more are gathered together. All you need are a few props, such as an old photograph, magazine, or trinket that has a story, and then begin to tell the story: "This is a picture of you and Dad on your wedding day. You are wearing your mother's wedding dress." Place the picture in their hand and let them hold it, then help them remember the story: "You had a bouquet of roses . . ." If you can give them a rose to smell at this point, you have used auditory, verbal, and tactile cuing, all of which are necessary to increase the chances that your message will be successful. Sit back and watch the magic moments unfold.

### Household chores can be fun together.

While there needs to be discretion in regard to the complexity of the task, allowing dementia patients to help you with certain chores such as dusting with a feather duster, wiping off the table, or putting the napkins out before dinner is not only an opportunity for success but it also gives one a feeling of self-worth. Practice this as frequently as one allows you to do so.

### Normalization time.

What was the person's routine for getting up each day? For going to bed at night? Did they do devotion in the evening with their family? Did they have a glass of orange juice and bowl of cereal every morning? If there was a particular habit that was routine and normal for the individual, try as much as possible to ensure these routines are *normalized* into their daily routine.

### *Sorting, stacking, folding, and snacking.*

Colored socks need to be matched. Assorted washcloths and hand towels need to be folded. The books need to be stacked. *Whew!* "We have worked really hard today. Would you like to join me for a snack? I have your *favorite*?" And that is when you pull out the pièce de résistance that is truly their favorite snack. Plus, we know it can be difficult to keep the calories high enough when dementia patients are in the pacing/wandering stages of the disease process. Helping persons living with dementia stay active, engaged, and participating in meaningful daily activities are excellent ways of bringing joy into the journey.

# Helpful Books and Websites

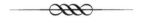

*Chicken Soup for the Soul: Living with Alzheimer's & Other Dementias* by Amy Newmark, ©2014

With 101 encouraging and inspiring stories by others like you, this book is a source of support and encouragement throughout your caregiving journey.

*Still Alice* by Lisa Genova, ©2008

*Still Alice* is a fictional story about the descent of a fifty-year-old university professor diagnosed with younger-onset Alzheimer's disease. The Alzheimer's Association assisted author Lisa Genova with her research, which included interviews with several members of past Early Stage Advisory Groups. The Association is also featured prominently in the book's plot. In addition, the Association worked with Genova to create the *Still Alice* discussion guide, specifically for people living with Alzheimer's. The guide, the first of its kind, is intended to help people with the disease use Alice's story to connect with their experience and explain it to others.

*Creating Moments of Joy Along the Alzheimer's Journey: A Guide for Families and Caregivers* by Jolene Brackey, ©2016

The new edition of Creating Moments of Joy is filled with more practical advice sprinkled with hope, encouragement, new stories, and generous helpings of humor. In this volume, Brackey reveals that our greatest teacher is having cared for and loved someone with Alzheimer's and that often what we have most to learn about is ourselves.

*Grandma and Me: A Kid's Guide for Alzheimer's and Dementia* by Beatrice Tauber Prior and Mary Ann Drummond, ©2017

A truly engaging yet informative book for young children on the topics of Alzheimer's and dementia. The beautiful artwork will capture children's attention, bring them into the story, and help them return on their own. *Grandma and Me* provides a gentle yet age-appropriate description of Alzheimer's disease, while providing tools that help children continue to have a relationship with their loved one despite the disease.

*Motherhood: Lost and Found* by Ann Campanella, ©2016

A sensitive, in-depth study of one woman's slow descent into Alzheimer's as detailed by her daughter, *Motherhood: Lost and Found* involves us in the dynamic of a multigenerational family as well as the author's own story: horses, poetry, three terrible miscarriages, and in her forty-first year, a final miracle.

Alzheimer's Association,
www.alz.org

Dementia Friendly America,
www.dfamerica.org

Alzheimer's Society (UK),
www.alzheimers.org.uk

Alzheimer Society (Canada),
www.alzheimers.ca

BrightFocus Foundation,
www.brightfocus.org

National Institute on Aging, National Institutes of Health,
www.nia.nih.gov/health/alzheimers

Family Caregiving, AARP,
www.aarp.org/caregiving

Center for Medicare Advocacy,
www.medicareadvocacy.org

"Alzheimer's Disease and Financial Planning," Web
MD,
www.webmd.com/alzheimers/guide/financial-planning#1

Angel Tree Publishing,
www.angeltreepublishing.com

"The Forgetting: A Portrait of Alzheimer's,"
www.pbs.org/program/forgetting/

This Caring Home,
www.thiscaringhome.org

# Alzheimer's Care Recipe

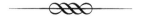

Ingredients:

2 cups of understanding

1 cup of knowledge

1 teaspoon of love

12 ounces (1 bag) of hugs and support

Directions:

Gently combine understanding and knowledge together on low speed. Mix in love at medium speed until mix becomes light and fluffy. Fold in hugs and support. When complete, drop teaspoon-sized servings onto a well-greased cookie sheet and bake in a warm, caring, and supportive setting 24/7 until a cure for Alzheimer's disease is found.

# About the Author

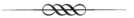

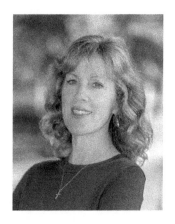

Mary Ann Drummond, RN, is a dementia educator, speaker, and author of titles including *Meet Me Where I Am: An Alzheimer's Care Guide, I Choose to Remember,* and co-author of *Grandma and Me: A Kid's Guide for Alzheimer's and Dementia.* Mary Ann has a passion for presenting innovative and successful strategies in both caregiver and provider settings to assist individuals with dementia so they may "live their best" each day. With over thirty years of nursing experience and sixteen years as a VP in the assisted living industry developing programs for dementia care, she credits much of her expert knowledge to the greatest teachers of all—individuals living with Alzheimer's disease and related dementias. A native of North Carolina, Mary Ann enjoys spending time with her family and working with organizations across the country to increase successful outcomes in dementia care.

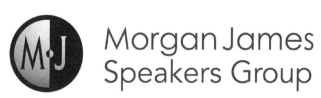

# Morgan James
# Speakers Group

www.TheMorganJamesSpeakersGroup.com

We connect Morgan James published
authors with live and online events
and audiences who will benefit
from their expertise.

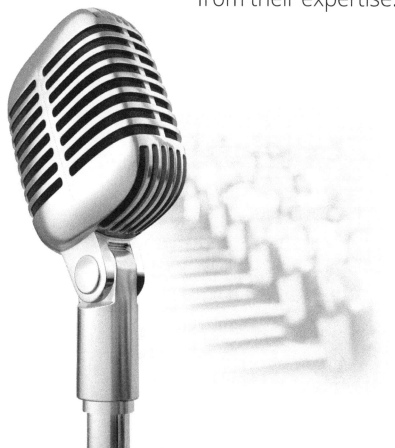

www.ingramcontent.com/pod-product-compliance
Lightning Source LLC
Jackson TN
JSHW080201141224
75386JS00029B/977